If, like many women, you feel you want to be physically fitter, that you could benefit from enhanced energy and increased self esteem, then perhaps running is something you should consider seriously. It requires very little in the form of specialist equipment, training or experience and the returns are almost immediate.

Alison Turnbull, contributing editor of *Running* magazine, started running in 1978. Inspired, like many others, from watching the 1981 London Marathon, she ran her first marathon in 1982, but prefers running short, fast races 'for fun'.

In 1983, concerned that not enough women were sharing the benefits of running, she launched the 'Sisters Project' in *Running* magazine, linking experienced women runners with those who wanted to run, but needed encouragement and information to start. This has proved enormously successful, and so far over 5,000 women have been encouraged through the 'Sisters' project.

This book is based very much on the practical experience of the author and those women with whom she has shared the experience of running. For any woman already running, or contemplating taking up this invigorating pastime, Running Together will prove invaluable.

RUNNING TOGETHER

RUNNING TOGETHER

Alison Turnbull

London
UNWIN PAPERBACKS
Boston   Sydney

First published in Great Britain by Allen & Unwin 1985.
First published by Unwin Paperbacks 1986.

UNWIN® PAPERBACKS
40 Museum Street, London WC1A 1LU, UK

Unwin Paperbacks
Park Lane, Hemel Hempstead, Herts HP2 4TE, UK

Allen & Unwin Australia Pty Ltd
8 Napier Street, North Sydney, NSW 2060, Australia

Unwin Paperbacks with the
Port Nicholson Press
PO Box 11–838 Wellington, New Zealand

Copyright © Alison Turnbull, 1985, 1986

ISBN 0 04 796129 5

Printed in Great Britain by
William Clowes Limited, Beccles and London

Dedication
To my father Tony (1916–1984) who fostered in his dumpy
daughter a love of sport in all its colours.

Contents

Acknowledgements

All the women (those who feature in the book and those too numerous to mention) who have helped other women enjoy the benefits of running; Dr Cindy Fazey, who asked all the right questions; Dr Beverley Kane, whose advice will help many runners to produce fit babies; and Lynne Butler, who made some very dull clerical work come to life.

While actively promoting the idea of women helping other women, I have never fought shy of asking men for help. I am particularly grateful to my editor at *Running*, Andy Etchells, and my husband, Robert Parry. Dr Hugh Bethell, Geoffrey Cannon, Steven Downes, Nicholas Keith, Dr Craig Sharp, Tony Ward and Derek Wyatt all provided inspiration and expert advice at various stages.

My own Big Brothers, Chris and Andrew Turnbull, actively encouraged my transition from spectator to runner, and I thank the women and men of Serpentine, Stragglers, and Wimbledon Windmilers running clubs for fuelling my enthusiasm.

Thanks are also due to Eileen Langsley, who took the photographs and to Louise Barton for the cartoons.

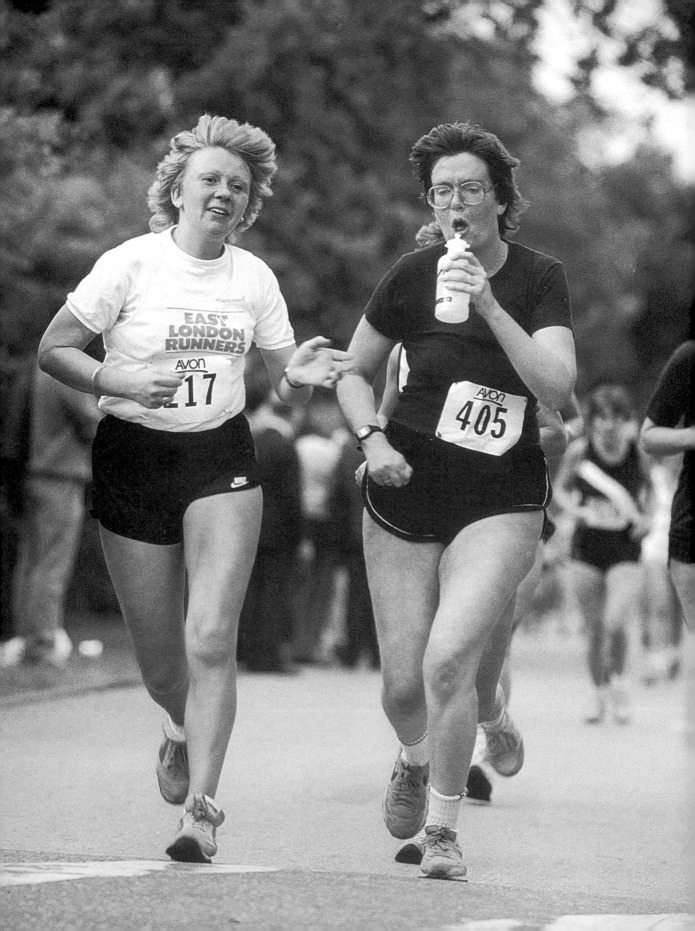

Foreword

This is a wonderful book – and timely. More and more women run now than ever before. And anyone taking those first tentative steps into the daunting world of exercise would do well to keep it as a constant companion.

From the profiles of newly converted runners with their breezy enthusiasm, to detailed advice on how to go about it, Alison Turnbull offers tips on not just how to start running, but, crucially, how to keep going.

Different people run for different reasons – increased stamina, more energy, weight loss, or simply that indefinable sense of well-being that follows naturally from it. But at the end of the day, these come down to one thing. Changing your life. This sounds a little sweeping. But to start running is to make a positive statement both to yourself and the world around you that from now on you will be stronger, fitter, and more confident both physically and psychologically. I wish when I had started running that I'd had such a sympathetic, sensible and FUN book to guide me on my first hesitant steps. It's one that is positively brimful with advice. Take it. You won't regret it.

Pamela Armstrong

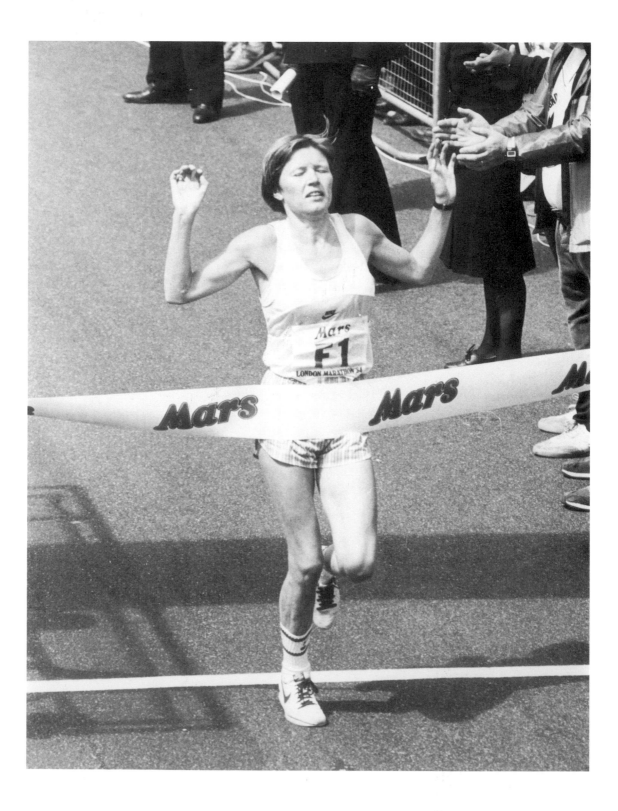

CHAPTER ONE
If *she* can do it, *I* can!

I started *running* on 30 March 1981, the day after the first London Marathon. Before that, I was a lumpy, halfhearted, fairweather jogger who got into shape once a year just enough to complete the two and a half mile *Sunday Times* National Fun Run without stopping.

My brother Andrew was accepted to run that first London, and I thought it would be fun to go along and watch. It wasn't fun at all. It was a dull, drizzly day, ideal for the runners but pretty miserable for the spectators. I tried to spot Andrew at several points along the course, but failed at most of them. I had a bad dose of 'marathon-watcher's eyeball' – if you've ever watched a big event like this you'll know what I mean! You stare for hours at the hordes of strangers rushing by, but you can't see your nearest and dearest even when they're right under your nose. Cold and wet, I descended into Tower Hill tube station swearing that it must be easier to *run* the marathon than to watch it. The next year I put this theory to the test and yes, running was a lot easier.

Only 300 women (in a field of 7,500) ran that first London Marathon. They were not just elite athletes running the 26 miles, 385 yards in under three hours (a time that takes a lot of talent and dedication) but women of all shapes, sizes and abilities.

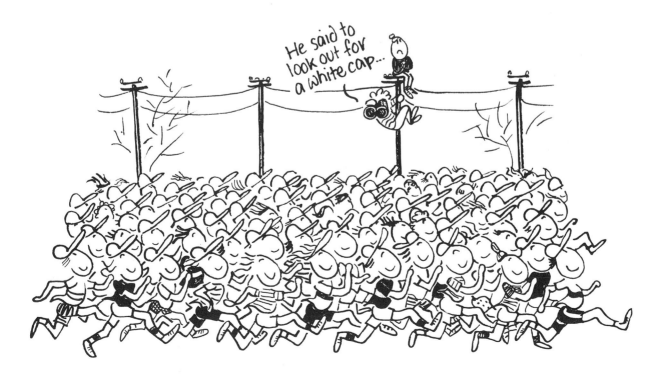

The winner of the women's race was Joyce Smith, who on that day became the first British woman ever to run the marathon faster than 2½ hours. Joyce, then 43, and the mother of two girls, had been an athlete all her life – she had her first taste of international competition in 1960 and captained the women's track team in the Munich Olympics in 1972. Her experiences were different, and rather remote, from other women of her age. But she showed wives and mothers in their middle years that a woman is by no means over the hill when she turns 40. Quite the reverse, in fact, for it was not until she was 41 that Joyce ran her first marathon and discovered the event for which she will be best remembered.

However, there were also women like Diana Cook from Isleworth, whose progress I had followed enthusiastically in the *Observer* newspaper. Di was a 'guinea pig' in a scheme hatched up by London Marathon Director Chris Brasher to train people of all abilities to run the marathon. I had taken a particular interest in her progress – she was the same age, had the same interests and started off from the same jogging baseline as I had. What I found most encouraging was that the schedules she was following in the *Observer* looked realistic. I tried some sample weeks, completed them and realised I could probably keep going if I had a target to aim for.

Then there was a 64-year-old Scot, Madge Sharples, who had started running 2½ years earlier. Madge jogged along quite happily at the back of the field, waving and chatting to everyone and she became a TV star overnight.

To my mind, those 300 women set women's running on its feet in this country. Women like me, soaked on the sidelines, and women at home glued to the TV, saw the likes of Madge Sharples and Di Cook, and said to themselves: 'If *she* can do it, *I* can!'

Diana Cook (The Guardian)

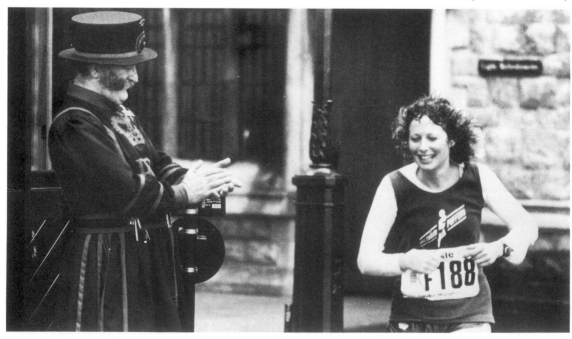

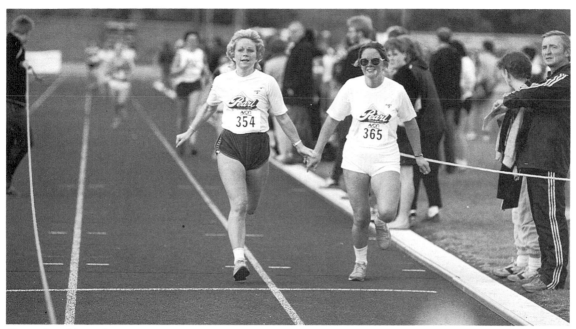

Running Together

If you think you're too fat, too old or too slow to start running or you're just not the sporty type, just get yourself out to watch one of these big events. You're sure to find some courageous old dear who is fatter, older and slower than you. Does she look ridiculous? Well, yes, perhaps her bottom or boobs are a bit wobbly – but does she look as though she cares? I'll bet she doesn't. In fact, even if she is tagging along behind a field of serious competitors she is the one with the widest smile and the warmest heart.

Sheila Giles is 54. As a child, she had a bone disease in her left leg and went to a school for crippled children. She started running when she was 52 and in that same year completed the Avon 10-mile race, a national championships in which the top woman can expect to finish in around 55 minutes. Two years in a row, she has rolled in last, and taken two hours and 11 minutes – more than twice as long as the winner. She runs with a pronounced limp, and can't run a mile in less than 11 minutes. On both occasions, she has finished to tumultuous applause, smiling and waving all the way. Now, if Sheila Giles can do it, *anyone* can!

I want you to meet some other women who run. Women with whom you can identify – as I did with Di Cook – and say, 'Oh yes, that's like *me*!' (Di and I are good pals now, and we're not, in fact, that similar – but it was the things we had in common that got me committed to regular running.)

These women can help you, because, as 54-year-old Betty Mackinnon from Glasgow says, 'Only someone who has been unfit and overweight can know the bliss of reversing the physical failings.' They are happy to pass on their experiences to you.

What makes these women tick? What athletic background (if any) did they come from? What did running feel like the first time around? How on earth do they fit running in with their work, their families, their lives?

PROFILES
NO MORE LEG PULLING

VICKY, 17, SCHOOL STUDENT WITH SATURDAY JOB, STAFFS.
Started running: 1981.
Now running: 45 miles a week.

At school: Running isn't taken seriously. I won our local cross-country league but my PE teachers weren't bothered — they didn't contact me to put me into races.

First run: I couldn't run for ¼ mile without stopping to catch my breath. I used to get my leg pulled by classmates, but now they have started taking my running seriously and some have even asked my advice on getting started.

Benefits:
★   more confidence in myself;
★   a goal to work for;
★   I have met so many nice people;
★   at my age I feel that I still have room for improvement, and so train harder.

Fitting running in with life: When I'm on holiday from school I run a long run in the morning and a short run at night. I cannot run on Saturdays as I'm on my feet all day working and find I'm too tired to run in the evening. When I'm at school I like to run before going to school and take a longer run in the evenings. Two nights a week I go to an athletics club and so only run in the evenings.

Other sports: orienteering, cycling.

FITTER FOR OTHER SPORTS

JANE, 18, SCHOOL STUDENT, KENT.
Started running: 1982.
Now running: 4½ hours a week, when school work and exams permit.

At school: I enjoy all sports. My PE teacher says I'm good, and thinks I'm quite good at hockey. As I hope to be a PE teacher, I need to try to have a good all-round standard in a variety of sports.

First run: The first time I went running 'out of school' I thought everyone was looking, and felt quite self-conscious, but then I realised joggers had become quite a common sight and I felt OK.

Benefits:
- ★ greatly increased my confidence. Because I'd been out running and didn't mind being seen out running, I did some training during the second half of the winter for school cross-country. This paid off, because I ended up running for London in the English Schools Cross-country Championships in March 1984;
- ★ running has improved my stamina for other sports.

Fitting running in with life: I try to run in the evenings when I don't have too much homework or revision for exams. This means that towards the summer my running practically ceases, then gets going again in the summer holidays.

Other sports: swimming, badminton, hockey.

'SUCH A WEED'

CHRISTINE, 24, CIVIL SERVANT, ESSEX.
Started running: 1983 (doctor's orders!).
Now running: Two hours a week.

At school: I was pretty useless and got a lot of stick from the girls in my class, but the teachers used to encourage me. I suppose they realised that I was doing my best considering I was such a weed. I couldn't even *lift* the shot, let alone 'put' it anywhere!

First run: I didn't worry about what people would think.

Benefits:
- ★ I feel better mentally on the days I run;
- ★ I sleep better. Before, I found that when I went to bed my mind ran riot — thinking about this and worrying about that. When I run, because I run like a zombie, all these thoughts come out, so I don't get all in a tizzy when I go to bed;
- ★ good for my figure. I still only weigh around 7½ stone, but I have a bit of shape now instead of being like a pole! I don't mind wearing short skirts and skimpy tops — I used to worry about knobbly knees and bony shoulders;
- ★ I have met a new boyfriend through running — and haven't looked back!

Fitting running in with life: I live at home with my parents, so it is easy to run in the evenings. It doesn't interfere with my social life either, because I drag my boyfriend round with me at least one night a week.

'PRIDE IN EVERYTHING I DO'

NICKY, 22, INTERIOR DESIGNER, CUMBRIA.
Started running: summer 1982, to use up free time at art college.
Now running: five hours a week.

At school: Gym never appealed to me, though I enjoyed hockey and cross-country (in which I was always near the back). I was never known as an athletic child — slightly overweight, I always felt self-conscious about games.

First run: Ran over the back fields at college (with no-one watching). Covered 1½ miles in 20 minutes! (A year later I ran a marathon in 3:48.) To start with I felt fat and unfit, but it hurt less as my training increased and weight decreased.

Benefits:
★ improved my figure (I have the confidence to wear a bikini now);
★ made more aware of what I eat, how I cook it, prepare it and serve it;
★ I have more confidence, and I've generally become a more out-going person;
★ life has meaning;
★ I seem a happier, healthier person;
★ I require less sleep;
★ I can sustain long, arduous hours of work;
★ I rarely lose my temper;
★ it has calmed my whole personality;
★ I have made new friends, from fun runners to serious athletes;
★ it gave me the confidence to go and teach outdoor pursuits to groups of children — something I would never have had the courage or the fitness to do before;
★ I take pride in everything I do.

Fitting running in with life: My highest running mileage (55 miles a week) was easily fitted in with my student life. Since I started work I need to fit it in on my day off, or run after work between 8–9.00pm. On Sundays I usually cycle as well. I manage to swim once a week now, which I know helps my breathing. It is difficult to go out on dark evenings, but I find once I get out there I enjoy it. Once I've reached the half-way mark, I find my pace increases, as I look forward to a hot shower afterwards!

Other sports: swimming, hill walking, cycling.

'I'VE LOST THREE STONE'

ANNE, 24, HOSPITAL THEATRE TECHNICIAN, CLWYD.
Started running: 1981, weighing 13st 7lb (5ft 2in).
Now running: 40–50 miles a week.

At school: I never used to turn up for PE lessons – my PE teacher thought I'd left school in form three!

First run: I felt embarrassed, but determined to get somewhere.

Benefits:
★ I've lost over three stone in weight . . . ;
★ . . . and gained a few tons of self-confidence;
★ clear skin;
★ a more relaxed attitude to life.

Fitting running in with life: I make time during dinner breaks and before work, if need be. I have to do at least two 'on calls' per week. When I'm not on call I usually run in the evening.

Other sports: squash, badminton, swimming, weight training.

FIT FOR EMERGENCIES

LIZ, 30, HOSPITAL DOCTOR, MIDDX.
Started running: 1983, seriously. Before that, spasmodic jogger.
Now running: 3½ hours a week.

At school: I used to be last in races with the class fatty, although I was thin, and poor eye-hand co-ordination made ball-games difficult.

First run: I thought I'd never be able to do much – once I'd run my first mile I was delighted.

Benefits:
★ when running regularly I smoke fewer than 10 cigarettes per week;
★ my body moves better, without wobbling;
★ I have more energy at work and can rush to emergencies without arriving breathless;
★ the main thing is a sense of satisfaction at being able to do something I would never have expected to be able to do.

Fitting running in with life: I run in the evening after work. I have no children, so it fits in well.

'SQUASHED PEAS ON THE HALL FLOOR'

EUGENIE, 30, JOURNALIST, DERBYSHIRE.
Started running: August 1982.
Now running: nearly four hours a week.

At school: I was absolutely useless at EVERYTHING! Furthermore, I loathed everything. I wanted to play football, but even at a trendy co-ed, this was a no-go area for girls. We had several PE teachers, none of whom noticed I was alive, except for one who used to pick on me in tennis lessons because I wore sunglasses to keep chronic hay fever at bay. She was a mega-cow! My chief recollections are of squashed peas on the hall floor (PE shared with morning assembly and school lunch) and the randy odd-job man having a good butchers up our gymslips. By puberty my mother quite happily helped me by supplying 'Eugenie has a period' notes about three times a month.

First run: I felt deeply inadequate! It brought back a lot of uncomfortable memories, but I suppose maturity helped me overcome them. I gave up the first time I tried, but persevered the second time, and really have stuck with it.

Benefits:
★ proved that I'm not the physical disaster school led me to believe;
★ my lungs are a constant reminder of a stupidly misspent 20s (30 fags a day), but I'm about 100 per cent fitter than I've been since I was about 11;
★ I enjoy running — not every run, but the general sensation and condition of running;
★ I think I might come to quite like my body after all.

Fitting running in with life: I work a four-day week, so there's no problem fitting running in. I generally go out at about 10.30am on the days when I'm working (I start work at 4.00pm) and mid to late

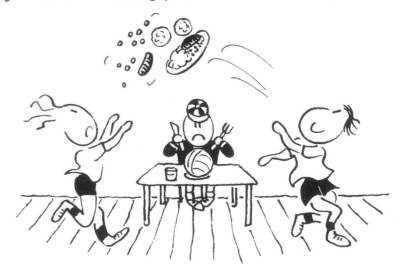

'GAWKY ASTHMATIC'

LYNNE, 30, ADMINISTRATOR, ESSEX.
Started running: 1983.
Now running: 30 miles a week.

At school: The class joke! I used any excuse (and as an asthma sufferer I could always summon up a wheeze) to avoid PE, and when I had to join in I deliberately messed about and made the most of my inadequacies.

First run: Awkward, embarrassed, fat, wheezy, sweaty, positive I wouldn't keep it up.

Benefits:
* ★ I find runners are friendly and trusting people;
* ★ I have become aware of my own responsibility for my health;
* ★ a run in the evenings after work makes all the petty problems disappear, and I now fit in a run *before* work if I have an important meeting or a difficult day ahead;
* ★ I joined Essex Ladies Athletic Club and it has turned out to be the best thing I could have done. Imagine how proud my parents are to think that their gawky, asthmatic daughter trains alongside members of the British Olympic team!
* ★ my asthma is under control. I can now run all distances without medication and I am able to leave my inhaler at home. This has boosted my confidence enormously. Now, whenever I feel a wheeze coming on I don't automatically reach for the inhaler — I try to relax and overcome it.

Fitting running in with life: I am not really organised to run to and from work or in the lunch hour — but it has been known! Usually I get home about 6.00pm, change and go out before I have a chance to change my mind. At weekends I run earlier in the day, quite often with my boyfriend. I am single and live on my own which makes things easier.

Other sports: swimming, Jane Fonda workouts.

afternoon on the days I'm not. However, I don't function too well before midday. In the winter I'll go out at around 3.00pm on days off. Long runs are usually saved for Saturday or Sunday. From time to time runs have to be missed because of appointments, but not too often.

Other sports: swimming, ski-ing.

'BREATHING SPACE'

LESLEY, 33, MOTHER, WORCS.
Started running: 1983, having had no exercise since the birth of daughter Lucy in 1981.
Now running: 2½ hours a week.

At school: I enjoyed PE and won colours for netball.

First run: I felt terrible. I've never smoked in my life, and considered myself to be fairly fit as I walk a lot, but I couldn't stop coughing for about two hours!

Benefits:
★ I've made friends;
★ I'm not so uptight;
★ I sleep much better;
★ running give me 'breathing space' — after a day with a toddler comes seven o'clock, freedom out running when no-one can get to me, no 'Mummy, Mummy!'
★ I still weigh about the same as I did before, but it doesn't wobble around half as much as it did;
★ I've achieved something. I stand on my own merit, not because I'm 'Mike's wife' or 'Lucy's mum' but because I'm me.

Fitting running in with life: I run with a friend in the evenings as I have no-one to look after my daughter during the day. My husband baths her and puts her to bed while I run — then he goes running.

'RUNNING MEANS THAT I CAN EAT'

MARY, 32, MOTHER, MIDDX.
Started running: 1981, after seeing first London Marathon.
Now running: 4½ hours a week.

At school: PE was good at my school. I would have enjoyed it more if I had not been a stone overweight, but I was in the netball and tennis teams. I can't remember doing much athletics, it was something you tried after school hours.

First run: I felt pleased with myself. I quite enjoy people looking at me. I don't mind being stared at, because I know I'm doing something a lot of people can't.

Benefits:
★ running means that I can eat. I'm a snacker — I eat four small meals a day with perhaps cake or biscuits mid-morning plus at least three apples a day. I couldn't eat all that lot if I didn't run!
★ I like getting out on my own — as soon as I'm out of the door I don't give the children another thought;

★ I enter the same races as my husband because I want people to know I run as well.

Fitting running in with life: I usually run in the evenings at about 7pm and my husband goes out when I come back. One long run a week, usually Sunday mornings (2–2½ hours). My husband looks after the three children (aged four, three and 18 months) while I'm out and vice versa. When we are trying to increase mileage, we take turns at going out at 6.30am (he has more turns than me!). Surprisingly we fit it all in very well. We usually relax for the evening together at about 9.00pm, by which time all the children are in bed. We usually go to bed at about 11.00pm.

Other sports: None apart from walking to and from school and shops and sometimes cycling to shops with the baby on the back of the bike.

'WARM GLOW OF SATISFACTION'

CAROL, 34, STAFF NURSE, MOTHER, NORTHUMBERLAND.
Started running: August 1982.
Now running: 35 miles a week.

At school: cross-country consisted of going to my friend's house for a quick cup of tea and joining in again as everyone approached the school. My teacher was very unsympathetic and made no attempt to find a sport that might suit us instead of bullying us into doing something we hated.

First run: I felt terrible — as if my lungs would burst and my legs would break. I also remember the pain of my bottom wobbling up and down.

Benefits:
★ at last there is something I can do — not brilliantly, but well enough to leave a warm glow of satisfaction;
★ I had a real hang-up about my body but running has made me look so much better;
★ I gave up smoking the first week I started — it just wasn't compatible with running.

Fitting running in with life: I work three full shifts per week. On work days I run during my lunch break (great for avoiding stodgy hospital food) and may do a short run in the evening. On my days off I like to run during the day and leave the evenings free — I think it's unfair on the children if both parents run in the evening.

Other sports: keep fit at the local sports centre.

FIGHTING THE FLAB

BARBARA, 36, PE TEACHER, MOTHER, HANTS.
Started running: 1982.
Now running: nearly two hours a week.

At school: It's such a long time ago! I enjoyed team games because I was fairly successful. 'Athletics', I seem to remember, covered high and long jump and 100yd sprints plus the odd egg and spoon race or sack race for sports day.

First run: Being the 'PE type' I thought I'd be fitter than I was — I'm wiser *now!*

Benefits:
* ★ I can share one of my husband's interests;
* ★ I find it a good and fairly cheap way of keeping fit;
* ★ there are good days and bad days. The good ones are when you go out feeling mentally and physically tired (not in the mood for running at all) but by some miracle you come back refreshed and with a sense of achievement;
* ★ it helps fight the flab — I don't have to worry about what I eat.

Fitting running in with life: In term time my elder daughter is at school and the younger one at play school two mornings a week, so I can run then if teaching preparation permits, otherwise it means running when my husband comes home in the evening. He's sympathetic, being a runner himself.

Other sports: badminton, aerobics.

'MENTALLY AGILE'

SUSAN, 34, MANAGING DIRECTOR, LONDON.
Started running: 1983, weighing 12 stone.
Now running: 20–30 miles a week.

At school: I went to school in New Zealand where sport is revered. I was a sprinter and also ran cross-country. House teams competed regularly, and competition was always regarded as important and a great source of pride.

First run: I could hardly make it to the end of the road, but I knew I wanted to continue, and I'm glad I did.

Benefits:
* ★ I lost nearly a stone in just over a year. Not a lot — but it stayed off, and I haven't dieted at all;
* ★ I've met some nice people through running;
* ★ I feel so much better physically;
* ★ I feel more mentally agile. I sleep better, wake up in the mornings bouncing and ready to go rather than having to drag myself up to face the world;

★ when you tell someone that you are going to run a 10-mile race, a marathon or whatever, even just a two-hour run on a Sunday and they react in horror, 'You? You'll never do *that!*' . . . the satisfaction when you've done it is pretty hard to beat.

Fitting running in with life: With difficulty! Although I live on my own, I am always out and about or entertaining, or working late, and I can't promise myself to be in any one place at any one time on a regular basis. So I have got into the habit of hoisting myself out of bed an hour earlier and running in the morning. Much to my surprise I enjoy it, although there are some evenings when I just know I want to go for a run, but I can't because I have other commitments.

Other sports: Swimming, walking and, till recently, cycling. I would love to do *much* more, but time is the problem.

BACK TO BOOKS

SYLVIE, 37, PART-TIME LECTURER/PART-TIME STUDENT, MOTHER, HERTS.

Started running: 1983.

Now running: 2½ hours a week.

At school: I was an athlete at school, but on leaving found it impossible to continue. It wasn't 'socially acceptable' for girls to run round the streets in those days! My PE teacher was not bothered about athletics and didn't like me as I hated hockey.

First run: I felt foolish and shattered yet determined to recapture the pleasure I used to get from it.

Benefits:
★ the fact that I disciplined myself to train regularly was influential in my decision to return to study after 15 years. I thought if my body could be disciplined, so could my mind;

★ I am more selfish — determined not only to be cook, chauffeur and cleaner but to do the interesting things *I* want to do — as the rest of the family do!

Fitting running in with life: My husband is very helpful with the children and cooking. He's also a lecturer, so he works varied hours and has time off in the day. Now both children have started school, we have had some runs together. I find it important to run on days when I have no commitment outside the home, as it is a good stress reliever.

Other sports: squash, keep fit, aerobics.

'MIDDLE AND FATTEST DAUGHTER'

KAREN, 37, TEACHER, MOTHER, BERKS.
Started running : 1982.
Now running: three hours a week.

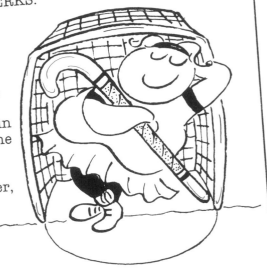

At school: I loved trampoline and dance, but loathed gym — I couldn't climb a rope and had no sense of balance. I hated all running about in netball and tennis, but was in the hockey team for four years as goalie. My father introduced me as 'my middle and fattest daughter, the goalie of the 1st XI. Do you know why she's so good? She's so fat, they can't get the ball past her.'

First run: Apart from feeling a fool (I went out at night so no-one would see me) I felt as if I had suddenly discovered a wonderful secret.

Benefits:
★ it sounds so corny, but running really has changed my life;
★ I now realise that I have not been 'fat' all my life, and at long last I don't feel negative about my body. I can accept it, warts and all. It feels good (I keep touching it in surprise) and I believe it will feel better;
★ I have more friends, and such a variety;
★ I feel 'whole' and well-balanced;
★ I used to say, 'I don't have an inferiority complex — I *really am* inferior.' For the first time in my life, I don't believe it.

Fitting running in with life: I try to run when I finish work at 12.00 because the children are at school. Evenings are difficult, with hobbies for the children, an evening meal, an irregular husband, and a car-sharing problem to contend with! We organise our runs fairly over the weekend.

Other sports: two weeks' ski-ing per year.

'I RESENT THE PLEASURE I MISSED'

DIANA, 38, CHIP SHOP OWNER, BRISTOL.
Started running: after London Marathon, 1982.
Now running: 20 miles a week.

At school: I can always remember the anxiety of the long jump, when I would wonder if I could even reach the sand pit! Only once did I not come last in a race. I was always the last one picked for any team. Teachers were absolutely unsympathetic. There was tremendous emphasis on winning — participation didn't count. I feel very resentful now of all the pleasure I have missed just because of other people's attitudes.

First run: I was apprehensive about my ability to go the distance — I never worried about the speed.

Benefits:
★ I started running with the sole purpose of running a marathon. After I had done it I felt ready to conquer Everest — I knew then that anything I really wanted, I could do;
★ I love the feeling of being fit;
★ when I am fit I rarely feel tired;
★ I am much more able to cope with my workload;
★ confidence — I started something over two years ago and I am still doing it — it's no flash in the pan.

Fitting running in with life: I run early in the morning. I used to stagger out of bed straight on to the streets, but I at least have a cup of tea first now — half an hour isn't going to make much difference.

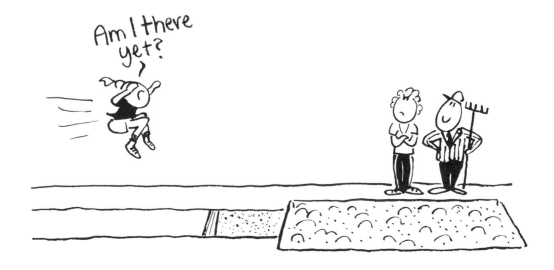

MOTHER AND SON IN HARMONY

MOLLY, 39, SCHOOL SECRETARY, GLOUCESTERSHIRE.
Started running: 1983.
Now running: four hours a week.

At school: I can only remember athletics being on the timetable for a week or so before sports day. Otherwise, we did a little gentle tennis, or country dancing in PE lessons. We did hockey in winter and I secretly quite enjoyed this.

First run: I felt foolish! I did not want to be seen, especially by pupils at the school where I work. I was also shattered to find how unfit I was.

Benefits:
★ I have lost about a stone in weight and maintained the loss;
★ I don't get as tired as I used to;
★ I feel I cope better under pressure;
★ my son is a very keen runner, and has always encouraged me to run. In turn I feel more able to help and support him and to take an intelligent interest in his running, which is probably the most important thing in his life at present (he is 16). Thus we have a common interest at a period when many mothers and sons experience friction and alienation. This is probably my greatest bonus!

Fitting running in with life: I have a full-time job and a family, so there are often times when my training session has to be scrapped. I was following a marathon training schedule of about 50 miles a week which was not only physically demanding, but also time-consuming. I was glad when a pulled muscle meant enforced rest, and during the lay-off period I decided to reduce my weekly mileage doing a few short runs and one long one.

A BETTER JOB

JOAN, 40, RECEPTIONIST/TELEPHONIST, SURREY.
Started running: 1983.
Now running: 2½ hours a week.

At school: I hated PE and took little or no interest. My sporting ability was pretty useless.

First run: I felt dreadful, mainly because I tried to run a mile first time out, and I couldn't — I had to stop about six times.

Benefits:
*   I am much more aware of my body and the need for a healthy diet — which helps to keep away the flab;
*   I have made new friends, mostly people like me who had ambitions to run a half-marathon but didn't really believe they could do it;
*   running has become a family thing, with my teenage son joining me on training runs;
*   I have more confidence to tackle other things. After running the Avon 10-mile race I knew that if I could do that, I could prepare myself for almost anything — and I found myself a good full-time job after doing uninteresting part-time ones for years;
*   I can cope better with job and family;
*   running gives me time to have my own thoughts. If I run alone the world's problems disappear and everthing is beautiful for a while.

Fitting running in with life: On Sunday mornings I get up much earlier than I used to, to do a long run. The two shorter mid-week runs have to fit in any time I can find the odd few minutes during the housework. Sometimes I go in my lunch hour from work.
Other sports: aerobics.

'REFUELLING MY SYSTEM WITH FRESH AIR'

LINDA, 40, MOTHER, PART-TIME SHOP ASSISTANT, ART TEACHER, WILTS.
Started running: 1979.
Now running: 20—40 miles a week.

At school: I did reasonably well, but sport was classed as a third-rate subject. No sport from leaving school at 15 to start of running career.

First run: I felt desperate! I started aged 35 and didn't expect to reach 36!

Benefits:
★ I have formed firm friendships;
★ freedom from domestic demands and chores;
★ fewer colds;
★ less mental strain;
★ lower heart rate (20 beats lower a minute);
★ a sense of personal achievement;
★ a chance to do something totally for myself;

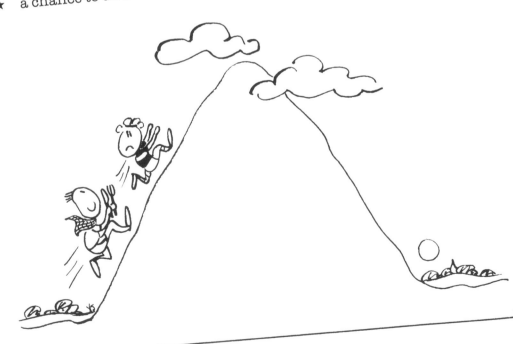

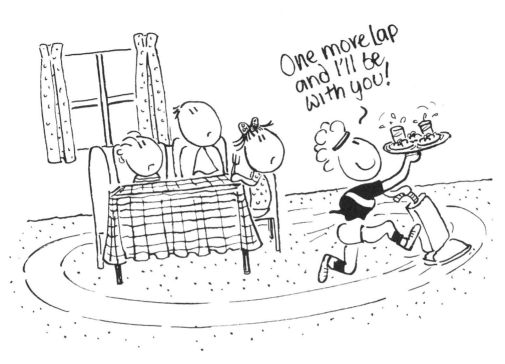

★ no pressures (unless you run with a husband who asks you what's for tea when you're struggling up a 1 in 4 hill!);

★ better sleep — most nights I hit the sack and know 'nowt' till morning;

★ refuelling my system with fresh air.

Fitting running in with life: After work: we are re-building a cottage 12 miles away, so I run all or part of the distance; After school: between vacuuming, dusting, moving engines and mixing mortar, feeding and cleaning cats, dog and horse.

Other sports: cycling, walking.

NEW FRIENDS AND NEW INTERESTS

MARION, 40, DEPUTY HEAD TEACHER, KENT.
Started running: 1981.
Now running: 40–45 miles a week.

At school: Games were for the non-academic — tennis a useful social asset.

First run: I felt sick.

Benefits:
* I feel younger than I did 10 years ago;
* I've stopped smoking;
* running a marathon was the best thing I've ever done — if I can cope with the pressure of that I can cope with *anything*.
* I'm psychologically stronger and totally unconcerned about what others think of me;
* I have far more energy and can do a lot more in a day than before;
* I have new friends, new interests, and a new awareness of the transitoriness of this life. It's the quality of life that counts — not the quantity;
* I enjoy meeting men as equals — though some still have hangups and have to win at all costs.

Fitting running in with life: I run to or from school twice a week; with a club on Wednesday evenings; and do a track session on Tuesdays. My husband runs and cycles, my son is 16 — so no baby-sitting problems! The housework is neglected, but no real hassle.

Other sports: swimming and cycling.

'I DON'T GIVE A DAMN'

CAROL, 40, SECRETARY, MOTHER, MIDDX.
Started running: 1981.
Now running: 30 miles a week.

At school: I avoided all forms of physical activity like the plague.

First run: I was shocked at how hard it was, and how out of condition I was, but I was determined not to let it beat me!

Benefits:
* weight loss (above a stone);

★ I now have confidence in myself due to a constant exposure to barracking, which I successfully ignore — I now don't give a damn for anyone's opinion of me;

★ if I am tired, cross or sad, a run will put it all in perspective for me.

Fitting running in with life: I get up at 6.15am, walk the dog, prepare breakfast for two children, coffee for me. Prepare school lunches, wake up children and husband, make beds. Leave home 8.00am. Return home 6.00pm, go out for run immediately, everything else can go to pot. Return feeling 100 per cent better, give children tea. In summer they play till late, so don't want food till 8.30-ish, which suits me as after my shower and exercise I can put the Hoover over the house and iron. In winter I feed the children first, do housework after. I usually end up eating about 9.00pm. At weekends I usually try to run for an hour in the early afternoon.

LIGHTER PERIODS

JUDY, 42, NHS SECRETARY, MOTHER, LONDON.
Started running: 1983.
Now running: four hours a week.

At school: I did anything I could to get out of sports. All the games mistresses were butch women in gymslips without any humour who favoured the sporty girls.

First run: I felt silly and exhausted over half a mile.

Benefits:

★ running has been the only thing I have achieved in years — it has given me a chance to accept a challenge at 40 and reach goals;

★ it has also salved my conscience at being unfit — I can justify excesses by saying 'at least I run';

★ I lost a stone after 22 weeks' running and maintained the loss;

★ since I was 13 I have suffered from painful, long, heavy periods. When I am training this is much alleviated — the single most important benefit for me.

Fitting running in with life: Running takes precedence over family commitments for both my husband and myself. However, I find it difficult after a hard day's work not to eat when preparing family meals and thus having to wait till very late at night before being able to run. It is not possible to run in the lunch hour — although I have changing and showering facilities it is an enormous upheaval mentally to adjust from the office desk to open road and back again.

'RUNNING HAS TRANSFORMED MY IMAGE OF MYSELF'

MAUREEN, 43, SOCIOLOGIST, RESEARCHER, MOTHER, KENT.
Started running: April 1979.

I had kept moderately fit over the years, but most of my sport was done alone. Then my husband entered the family in a 'fittest family' competition without telling us! One of the compulsory events was 1,000 metres cross-country. I had no choice — I *had* to go out and train.

First run: My throat burned, my legs felt like jelly. I was embarrassed at my podgy shape. I ran under cover of darkness — the race was my first run in daylight! It was a revelation — I came 10th out of about 40 women (and we were third family). I can remember the euphoria of achievement and also the hacking cough which lasted for half an hour afterwards.

Benefits:
- ★ my social life has expanded rapidly;
- ★ my self-esteem is increased — I *feel* good;
- ★ running has transformed my image of myself — now those who sneer at me from passing cars are only worthy of my complete indifference to them;
- ★ sometimes, on a training run or in a race, I *fly*. My legs and feet skim the pavement, I feel that I look like Kathy Cook or Seb Coe. Then it is all worthwhile — I hit a running high and feel strong.

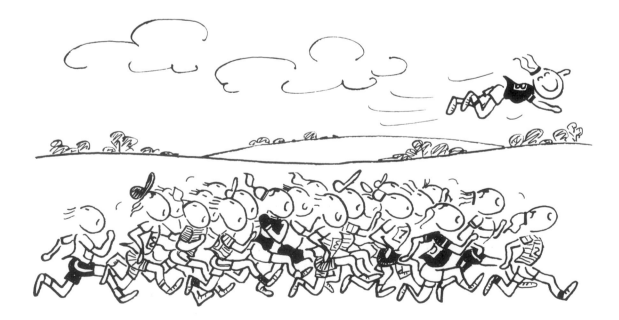

Fitting running in with life: All my family (husband, two sons, two daughters) run, so home life fits around running. Twice a week my daughters and I train with the club — dinner is eaten as late as 9.00pm on those nights. I've also trained early mornings as well as before work. Weekends are taken up with competition and long runs.

'I'D DIE WITHOUT IT'

JULIE, 52, SECRETARY, NIGHT SCHOOL TEACHER, LIVERPOOL.
Started running: 1981, after seeing first London Marathon on TV.
Now running: 20 miles a week.

At school: Unfortunately we didn't do athletics. I was very keen on cricket, and was carried off with concussion in the Aberdare Cup (lacrosse). My PE mistress always bawled at me to 'run *faster*' in both lacrosse and cricket.

First run: A friend put me down on the promenade at Otterspool and said, 'I'll meet you at the other end.' This was about half a mile, up and down the grass verges, while she kept to the winding promenade road above. When I reached the other end she wasn't there, so I jogged back again only to find that she had driven back to where we had started. In all I jogged about 1½ miles, and felt marvellous apart from being tricked into doing three times as much as I thought I could!

Benefits:
★ my figure has improved by 1½ stone less weight;
★ I feel and look younger;
★ I've gained confidence and can face the world much better — I seem to hold my head high!
★ I have made a whole lot more friends;
★ I used to be a bad sleeper, and was a very restless person. I used to take a sleeping tablet once a week or so, but now I very rarely take one — I can relax better without;
★ I had a hysterectomy about 10 years ago and now have a lot of 'hot flushes', but I don't notice them when I'm running.

Fitting running in with life: It's hellish difficult, but I'd die without it! I sneak out whenever I can when home from work. I have to play it by ear, because I must consider Mum, aged 86.

SCIATIC PAIN HAS GONE

BETTY, 52, MIDWIFE, GLASGOW.
Started running: 1983.
Now running: 2½ hours a week.

At school: PT was jerky exercises, touching toes and jumping over horse and box. I do not recall that I received any encouragement. I wore spectacles and was not allowed to wear them during PT. Being short-sighted did nothing to help my confidence or skill.

First run: Breathless! But after a time I was asking myself why it had taken me 50 years to discover that running was a pleasure.

Benefits:
★ an activity which my husband and I can share;
★ I have had less 'sick time' since starting running;
★ my weight is gradually going down;
★ I have been a migraine sufferer since 1969. I find that I can still go for a run even when my head is very painful;
★ I had sciatica which became more debilitating each year. About five weeks after I started running I was pain free for the first time in three years;
★ my muscle tone is much improved, my posture is better and I actually *have* muscles where previously there was flab;
★ I have a new lease of life;
★ I realise I will never break any world records, but the enjoyment I receive is out of all proportion to the amount of time that it takes!

Fitting running in with life: I work permanent night duty, so I run in the morning when the shift is over. When not working we are able to go out a little earlier. We look at my duties on a fortnightly basis and plan our running programme to fit in.

Other sports: keep-fit, yoga.

BEATING DEPRESSION

JOAN, 46, BAKERY PACKER, CHESHIRE.
Started running: 1983.
Now running: Nearly four hours a week.

At school: I was not very keen on sport — I pushed myself just enough to stop the teacher 'having a go' at me.

First run: I couldn't even run to the end of the avenue without stopping.

Benefits:

★ running gives me time to myself, either to think or just 'switch off' without anyone demanding my attention;

★ running seems to have stopped the 'hot flushes' of the menopause — apart from those caused by running itself, which I am quite happy to put up with;

★ running got me back into shape after my hysterectomy and took away the feeling that part of my life was over;

★ I have a marvellous sense of freedom with every run;

★ my depression was so severe at times that I felt suicidal and didn't want to go on. Now, if I put my running shoes on and get away from everybody and everything I can run it off or at least make it not so bad;

★ running is an easy cure to restlessness. I just run till I've no energy left to *be* restless;

★ after a fortnight of running I found out that I couldn't smoke and run as well. Then I suddenly found I wanted to run more than I wanted to smoke — so I stopped, and have never smoked since;

★ when I feel really wound up I run, and upsets, anger, frustrations all disappear and the world is lovely again.

Fitting running in with life: I run at 5.30 in the morning. This means I have time to get home and change before starting work at 7.30. When pushed for time I run to work (about five miles).

NO MORE COLD FEET

SHEILA, 47, SCHOOL MEDIA RESOURCES OFFICER, OXON.
Started running: 1979.
Now running: nearly four hours a week.

At school: Hard to remember! I was always keen, but we didn't have the variety of sport offered today — though everyone took part and seemed to enjoy it. We didn't play hockey as the field was used as an allotment after the war!

First run: I went out at night at first, but the further I ran the more confident I got, and then I went out in daylight at the weekend.

Benefits:
  ★ helps my circulation — I always used to have cold feet and hands;
  ★ a sense of achievement and well-being;
  ★ I'm hardly ever ill;
  ★ helps keep my weight steady;
  ★ it is a lovely experience running in Blenheim Park on a sunny morning — a good way to start the day.

Fitting running in with life: I get up early in the morning and go for a 20–40 minute run with my husband. My two sons are at college and I only have to cycle 500 yards to school where I work, so it fits in very well.

Other sports: tennis.

THE FOG HAS LIFTED

KATH, 47, HOUSEWIFE, MIDDX.
Started running: 1983.
Now running: Five hours a week.

At school: I attended a private convent, and hence played no sport at all, with the exception of netball — when a lay person could be found to supervise. All other PE very basic exercises and Scottish country dancing.

First run: Embarrassed! I felt certain everybody was looking at me!

Benefits:
  ★ life before running was like looking through glasses with the

lenses fogged up. I have totally altered my philosophy on life and solved a number of personal problems;

★ I am very aware — of my body, environment, what I eat, and other people;
★ I have 10 times more energy;
★ I have lost weight.

Fitting running in with life: I run early in the morning, which leaves the remainder of the day free.

Other sports: swimming, tennis, exercise class, occasional cycling.

'MY SEX LIFE IS MARVELLOUS'

LAVINIA, 47, SOLICITOR, MOTHER, BEDS.
Started running: September 1982.
Now running: 35 miles a week.

At school: Plenty of encouragement, although if you wanted to improve it was down to you. All stopped when I left school at 15. In those days there were not the facilities or encouragement to continue as there are today. I was a very good athlete and netball player.

First run: I felt very unfit and conscious of my legs and backside being too fat. I was concerned I might have a heart attack.

Benefits:
★ everyone has commented what a difference running has made to me;
★ it has made me more confident;
★ I have lost weight in the right places and feel much better for it;
★ I have more energy and mundane tasks don't get me down;
★ I don't get so tired;
★ I have met many new people;
★ I now have a lover and my sex life is marvellous.

Fitting running in with life: most of my running is done in the evening after work, and I often don't finish work till 7.00pm. I cook my evening meal after my run. Sometimes I run in the morning before going to work but this is usually when it is very warm.

Other sports: walking the dog when he doesn't run with me.

HOPELESS AT GYM

FRANCES, 49, CIVIL SERVANT, CLWYD.
Started running: regularly, 1983, with the dogs, in the Clwyd Hills.
Now running: four hours a week.

At school: I remember my gym mistress wailing hopelessly, 'You *look* as though you'd be good at gym, why can't you do it?' I may have looked right, but I was utterly hopeless. There was no athletics on offer in those days.

First run: I felt rather pleased! I'd heard someone who ran marathons say that when they started, they couldn't run a mile, so I thought I'd see if I could, and I could! So I could run marathons, too!

Benefits:
★ at my age, I have a much better chance of winning things than younger women — it's great fun;
★ I've joined the Deesside Athletic Club and met some marvellous people;
★ while you can run on your own, you do get to make a lot of friends, and running people seem so nice.

Fitting running in with life: Neither my work nor my home life have to be tied to set hours — no small children to care for, very easy going husband and son. I can partly work in the evenings, so I can run in the day.

Other sports: circuit training, long walks.

'COME ON, NAN!'

DAPHNE, 53, STATE ENROLLED NURSE, SUFFOLK.
Started running: August 1982.
Now running: 20–25 miles a week.

At school: So long ago! I was only good at hockey — hopeless at PE and never did running except in games.

First run: Short jog in park, followed by more short jogs, always when park was deserted! I felt shattered but determined to do better.

Benefits:
★   I feel happy and more healthy – life began at 50!
★   I have made many friends of all age groups;
★   my arthritis has improved greatly since I started running;
★   my life is interesting and full;
★   I have not lost much weight, but look a better shape;
★   in a race it was lovely to hear children calling out, 'Here comes my Daddy' – but it gave me even greater pleasure to hear two little boys say, 'Here's my Nan. Come on, Nan!'
★   there's a wonderful world out there in the sun, the fresh air, the rain, snow, wind, and I love it.

Fitting running in with life: I work night duty in 12-hour shifts, four one week, three the next. It's difficult to find the time and energy to run. I try not to have more than one day's rest at a time, even if I only do a very short run.

Other sports: swimming, cycling, Gym'n'Trim.

Are you convinced now? Who would have guessed that a simple activity like running could have so many physical, social and psychological benefits? No wonder so many more women are taking up running and sticking with it. Aren't these benefits that you want to reap, too? Let's look at some of them again:

Weight loss
Many women found that their weight stopped going up, and some lost weight – without dieting! They also became more aware of the foods they ate and more conscious of the need for a healthy, balanced diet. Later, you'll find out that your weight isn't the most important measure of your fitness.

Giving up smoking
Running and smoking don't really go together. Breathing takes oxygen and other gases from the air around you; your lungs absorb the oxygen into the bloodstream and your heart pumps oxygen-rich blood round the arteries. Your veins collect all the waste gas and take it back to the lungs for you to breathe out.

Smoking interferes with this process – like driving the wrong way down a one-way street. You inhale harmful gases that your body doesn't need. These gases take a free ride round the body in the arteries and limit the amount of oxygen you can take in. Women smokers taking up running suffered tightness in the chest and coughed more – and eventually decided they'd rather run than smoke.

More energy, not less
When you are fit, your heart doesn't have to pump so many times and your body is more relaxed about the work it has to do. In short, you're cruising along the motorway in fifth gear instead of chugging around town in first.

Better sleep patterns

When you are fit, you find you get far more done in the day than you could have hoped for before. If you go out for a run, you may be able to put your thoughts and worries into perspective. When you go to bed, you tend to fall asleep immediately, and when you wake in the morning your body feels as if it's been on holiday.

Question

PROJECT 1
WHO ARE YOU?

Throughout this book there will be Projects for you to tackle. Some will be active projects designed to help you move and learn about your body and to find out what it does when you exercise. Others are more relaxed — I'll simply want you to sit down and think and write about what you have done and how you feel.

You will need a simple ruled exercise book and a pen or pencil. The book will become your own personal Running Book to report on all the Projects you do. Later on it will become your first training diary and a vital record of your daily progress. A year from now you will be amazed at the progress you have made.

Good news. This project can be done sitting down — no exertions of any kind! I want you to look ahead and think about yourself in a year's time. Write a list of all the things about yourself you'd like to change. They could be physical things, like losing weight or giving up smoking; they could be social things, like making new friends, changing your job or learning a new skill; or they could be mental things, like being less irritable, less depressed or more confident. Whatever your age, do you think there's something in life that you have missed?

When your list is finished, I want you to go back over this chapter, especially the profiles. Is there someone here that you can identify with? Can *you* make the sort of changes that she has done? Can running help *you*?

Dig out, or have taken, a photograph of yourself — looking your oldest, fattest, spottiest, most awful. Stick it in your book as a reminder of the things you want to change.

The new you starts here.

Clearer skin and better circulation

When you first start to run, you will notice how red-faced you look afterwards. You will also sweat a little. This doesn't mean you're about to have a heart attack – quite the opposite. It shows that your body's thermostat, which keeps you cool when you are hot and warm when it's cold, is working normally. It also means that oxygen-rich blood is getting to every last blood vessel to take away the impurities and cleanse the skin from within – rather like a sauna bath. You may not like feeling red-faced immediately after a run, but wait till other people tell you how well you're looking! Running can make you feel good inside *and* make you look good from the outside.

Friendship

You can make friends with women and men from all walks of life and expand your horizons.

PROJECT 1
WHO ARE YOU?

I wonder sometimes. I'm Sue. I'm 38 and married to Jack, with three children — 9, 7, and 2½. I have a part-time clerical job at a small car hire company round the corner. I work more to meet people than for the money, which isn't wonderful. We're not too badly off, and for the most part, happily married.

Things I'd like to change

I smoke 30 a day — I'd like to give up. I'm about a stone overweight. I'm not *fat* but I *feel* fat.

I would love to be less ratty with Jack and the kids — but I always seem so tired and irritable. I'd like to widen my social life. All my friends are Jack's friends or mothers of the kids' friends. I'd like some friends of my own!

I want to set myself a target — and reach it! (Not dieting — I'm hopeless!)

Our first run!

Jill and I ran gently for about 5 minutes as far as the pillar box at the end of Windermere Road. Just as we were thinking it was easy, we ran out of breath. Jill started to walk, then me — so we walked/ran home. Disappointed that we didn't run all the way straight off, but quite pleased, anyway.

Back indoors, felt a bit 'choked' — tight neck, cough. Legs felt OK. All right after 10 minutes or so.

Still a big way to go.

Family life

Running is an activity you can share with your family – and it can improve your relationship with your husband and children.

Escape route

Running can also give you a chance to have some time to yourself away from family or work pressures. Some women use this time to let off steam about their problems, others use it as a time to switch off and forget them. My training sessions are creative periods in which I think about articles or chapters I am going to write, or in which I chat to someone else about the burning issues of the day, and usually pick up some bright ideas. Some people describe their daily run as a 'holiday'. Just think, if you can manage to run for three hours a week (the target I'll be setting you in Chapter 8) – at the end of the year, you'll have clocked up an extra *week's holiday*!

Achievement and pride

Whether you run for fitness or competition, you can set yourself goals. When you reach those goals, you'll be delighted with your achievements. Having achieved one goal you may think about other targets in your life that you'd like to reach – other things you've thought about doing, but always put off – like changing your job or taking an Open University degree.

Confidence

It's not easy to begin with and there are all manner of excuses you can make up for not wanting to be fit. One of them is that you'll worry about what other people think or say about you. But, once you have conquered your early fears and doubts, you'll be able to hold your head up high and never mind other people. This confidence can help you in other aspects of your life.

Body awareness

Running can help you to think positively about how your body works. You'll understand it better and know your own limitations. You'll take more interest in your diet, and think carefully about the good and bad things that you feed yourself each day. And you'll start to love your body, warts and all.

Identity

It's important you have your own identity – and that you don't think of yourself as probably somebody's secretary, mother or wife. It's very easy to fall into the trap of believing that other people cannot do without you. Running can help you think about the most important person in your life – you.

CHAPTER TWO
Excuses, excuses

Starting a new, healthy way of life is easy. Anyone can diet for a day, or go out for a single brisk walk. *Sticking* to your schedule, keeping your resolutions . . . that's the difficult part. It's so easy to find excuses not to run. Let's look at some of them.

'I'm too old'
New Yorker Gwen Clark is 93. One day when she was 86, she was sitting in Central Park watching the joggers milling past. She wanted to share their enjoyment. She started – not running, but race-walking, a brisk rhythmic exercise ideal for a woman her age. Now she walks seven miles a day. Fellow American Ruth Rothfarb started running at 72. At the age of 80 she ran a marathon in 5 hours 37 minutes.

It's never too late to start. However old you are, gentle exercise can give you a new lease of life, and shake off the blues that often come with retirement and advancing years.

'I'm too fat'
In 1982, Belinda Charlton, of Hampshire, was 21 stone and had just had a hysterectomy. She was extremely depressed. Like me, she watched a London Marathon and thought she'd like to have a go, though like Cinderella going to the ball, she reckoned her chances were pretty slim, because her body certainly wasn't.

But miracles do sometimes happen, and when her stepson suggested that Belinda should start running, it was just the magic wand she needed. She didn't dismiss the idea as totally ridiculous. After all, she had nothing to lose but her weight. To begin with, she went out in ordinary clothes and stout shoes (and carrying a handbag so that no-one would guess her secret!) and walked for 10 minutes a day, five days a week. Gradually she progressed to running, checking first to see that no-one was looking. She was still

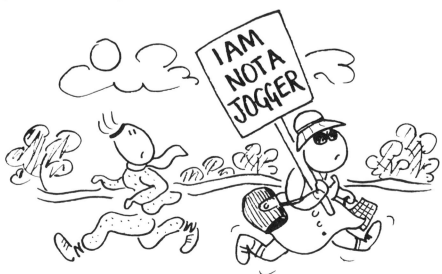

wearing her ordinary clothes – an important milestone was the day she left her handbag at home! Her confidence grew, and eventually she treated herself to a tracksuit. In her first year of running she lost over four stone, eating sensibly and taking more pride in her appearance. She started to train for the London Marathon, egged on by viewers of the local TVS television channel who followed her progress eagerly. In 1984, a trim 10 stone, she ran the London Marathon in 4 hours 25 minutes.

'I'm too decrepit'

Twenty-eight-year-old Linda Down from New York was born with cerebral palsy. She has to walk with crutches, her jelly-legs dragging behind her. In 1982, unemployed and at a low ebb, she started exercising, and, telling no-one except her twin sister Laura, entered for the New York City Marathon. At ten o'clock in the evening, when most of the other runners were dancing away their stiffness at post-marathon parties, Linda crossed the line in a triumphant 11 hours, 15 minutes. The following year, she completed the course in 8 hours, 46 minutes. Linda 'runs' for the same reason as any other woman – weight loss, feeling great, thinking clearly. But she has an extra challenge and the strength to fight her disability. And there's a bonus – her exercise has actually *strengthened* her spastic legs.

Freda Horrocks, 42, from Putney, has been blind since suffering a fall when she was only three. When Freda was 38 she took up water-skiing, where she met her boyfriend David Musgrove, who is also blind. David ran the London Marathon in 1984 with a sighted partner, Peter Felix. Although she couldn't see the occasion, Freda was enchanted by the atmosphere. She figured if David could do it, she could, and she enlisted the help of Peter Felix's wife Helena to be her guide as she trained for the 1985 London Marathon.

Patricia Nolan, 39, from Leeds, is an insulin-dependent diabetic. She runs up to seven miles three times a week 'without making a religion of it' and believes that running helps her to 'iron out the peaks and troughs of blood sugar levels'.

In February 1983, aged 45, Irene had a small cancerous breast-lump removed and afterwards she needed extensive radiotherapy. 'My whole world collapsed, and nothing seemed important or had meaning,' she says. Her sister persuaded her to start running. 'I had the choice of going home to die or starting to run,' she says.

The radiotherapists thought she was crazy. 'You won't cope – the treatment will knock you over,' they threatened, 'we'll find you lying in some gutter yet.' 'I was full of determination to succeed. I hadn't told my mother of my illness, and I was making sure I wasn't going to have to.'

To her doctor's amazement, Irene survived the treatment, and lost only one day from work. 'Even my closest friends do not suspect.' On the wall of the radiotherapy room, she says, there was a picture of a seagull in full flight, with the words beneath: 'I can because I think I can.'

And every week, I hear a new story of someone who has picked her/himself up from life's scrapheap and started running. There are women and men running with artificial limbs, with heart pacemakers, blind, deaf, dumb, deformed or mentally handicapped people. People, I'm sure, who are worse off than you are. Often, they run to raise money for others who are worse off than *they* are. These people make me feel very humble. Beside them, my own excuses pale into insignificance.

'I haven't got time'

Time is probably woman's most precious commodity, and you have to use it wisely. It is difficult for a mother with a job to find the time for regular exercise, but once she has done so, she is actually more likely to stick to her schedule than a younger, single woman without ties – who has plenty of other interests, and isn't worried about age creeping on.

Silvia, aged 33, has two boisterous young boys and is a full-time student. This is her typical day:

7.00 wake up, get boys ready for school, breakfast, tidying up
8.45 drive boys to school and myself to college
10–3.00 lectures
3.30 pick up Daniel from school
4.00 pick up Michael from day nursery
4–7.00 play with boys, read stories, talk about their schoolday, cook dinner, house-work, bath children and put them to bed
7–8.00 out for a jog, then shower
8–8.30 dinner
8.30–10.30 study and work for college
10.30 bed

Silvia has time. Like the women mentioned in the opening chapter she *makes* time to run, because that hour is an important break for her, a time when the children and the housework aren't making any demands on her. She has time to reflect on her college work, and to plan the day ahead. Her run is her daily 'holiday'.

'It's boring'

Running *can* be extremely boring, especially if you are running alone or with a dull companion who doesn't say much; and especially if you're pounding out the same old routes at the same old pace and you don't feel as if you're becoming any fitter.

'I'm afraid of being attacked'

Good. For with that fear comes common sense. There *are* weirdos about, in places where you don't expect them, and often in broad daylight. A would-be attacker depends on an element of surprise, so it makes sense always to have your wits about you.

Perhaps some of the common sense bears repeating.

★ Avoid isolated places. Now, if you followed this instruction to the letter, you'd miss out on 99 per cent of Britain's beautfiful running routes – the long-distance foot-paths, the canal towpaths, the city parks. The important thing is to find someone else to enjoy these places with, and to save your solo running for well-lit roads in residential areas.
★ Avoid running alone. This book is about running together – whether with women or men. If your husband or boyfriend is too fast or slow for you. find someone else who is prepared to run at your pace – perhaps someone who is older, or coming back from injury or, like you, is just beginning.

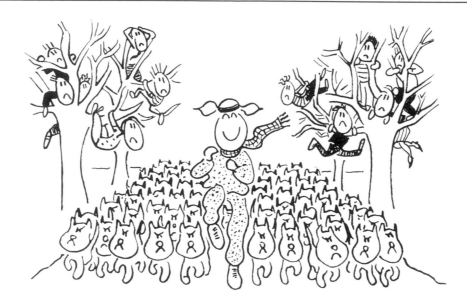

Or go out with the dog. In the USA, Shelley Reecher started a 'rent-a-dog' system, 'Project Safe Run'. After she was raped, Shelley started to run with her Dobermann pinscher and then found other women asking to borrow the dog. She bought a 'fleet' of the dogs and now hires them out regularly. Each carries a small backpack with emergency telephone numbers and change for the phone. None of the dogs has yet had to protect its temporary mistress. 'When you run with a Dobermann,' says Shelley, 'people just part like the Red Sea.'

Even the humble border collie can be woman's best friend. Jane Bird of Milton Keynes says she owes her running success to her border collie Shep, because she can run early in the morning and late at night in safety and thus fit her running in with her family and work. Sharon Payne from Birmingham is a nurse in an intensive care unit, and she bought her retriever, Barney, especially to run with at odd times of day.

★   If you *must* run alone, don't switch off. It's becoming quite trendy to jog with a personal hi-fi, so that there's just you and Mahler's Fourth or Dire Straits, or whoever turns you on. I think these small-scale cassette players are terrific, but not for running. Here's why. In the summer of 1984, a woman runner was raped in Richmond Park at 4.30 in the afternoon. She was running alone, tuned into her personal hi-fi. Consequently, she did not hear the tell-tale crackling of twigs, the heavy breathing . . . she couldn't act fast enough.

Apart from attack, on main roads you also run the risk of being run over. And London Marathon Director Chris Brasher tells the cautionary tale of the day he was miles away, well into Beethoven's Ninth, when he discovered he had gone too far down

Being wired up for sound is fine in a race, but be wary about running alone with a personal hi-fi.

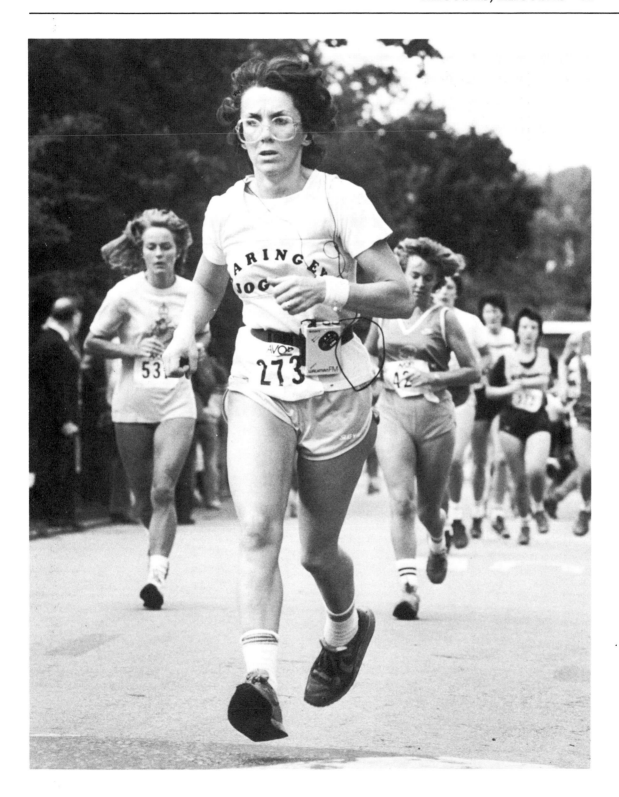

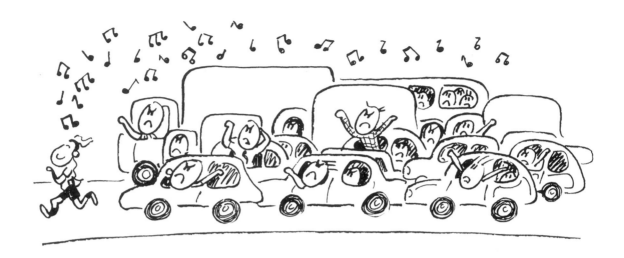

the towpath for his current level of fitness, and it was a struggle to reach home again. So, leave the personal stereo at home and sing to yourself, if you need to be entertained. Even if the attacker's not a rapist, he may still want to steal your stereo or jewellery, and he might hurt you in the process, so don't wear expensive jewellery.

★ *Do* always carry some kind of identification. The cheapest way to do this is to buy a dog tag and have it engraved with the name and number of someone to contact in case of emergency. This is particularly useful if you have allergies, a rare blood group, or want to donate your organs. Sorry to be so morbid, but if you *do* go under a bus when you're out running these simple precautions make life easier for other people.

★ Always tell someone where you're going, and for approximately how long.

★ If you're particularly scared, you can buy a small but loud alarm or whistle to hang round your neck, or carry a small aerosol – though don't hold me responsible if you use this in earnest on the wrong person!

I can't tell you what to do if you *are* attacked. Your own survival mechanisms and your instant summing up of the situation will tell you whether you're better off lying back and passively accepting your fate; trying to talk calmly to your attacker; or going for his eyes or his crotch.

If you hear someone coming up behind you, and you are suspicious of their motives, use the element of surprise. Take a deep breath, look at your watch, and suddenly cross the street or shoot off in a different direction. If you're in a residential area, it's dark and you're frightened, run up to a front door, ring the bell and pretend you live there. You may have some explaining to do, but this might just shake an attacker off your tail.

If the attack is inevitable, memorise everything about your attacker – features, clothes, accent, even smell – and *tell the police*. Bringing the man to justice may be difficult for you, but it's vital for other women.

'I'm afraid of being yelled at by motorists'

You can't win. Whether you're slim, leggy and suntanned, or pale with acres of unwanted flesh hanging out all over the place – you'll be yelled at. (I know – I've been both!)

It's often difficult to tell whether 'Get them knees up, darlin'' means

★ You're a very attractive woman whom I wouldn't mind seeing more of;
★ You're a very unattractive woman who shouldn't be out in the street looking like that;
★ I really admire what you're doing and wish I had the time/motivation/courage to go out and do it myself.

So it's difficult to know how to react. Although I've been guilty of it, I don't really think that sticking two fingers up and saying 'F*** off' really does anything for men's acceptance of women's running – and in some cases it may provoke and anger the guy. In others he will be laughing to himself because, essentially, he has won.

Just try to think of yourself as the winner. According to personality you can:

★ Smile sweetly, wave, say nothing, and run a little faster, just to show off. Particularly recommended if your big-mouthed friend is stuck in a traffic jam.
★ Ignore the abuse and, if it makes you angry, turn the anger inside – that'll make you run faster, too.

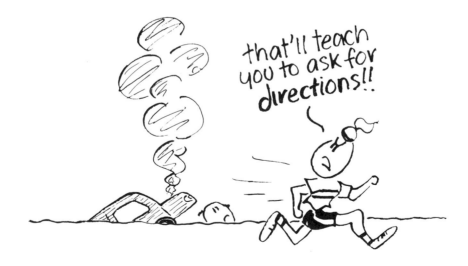

★ Think up something witty to say, like 'Shut up and eat your Yorkie Bar!' or 'If I picked my knees up, I'd fall over.' This is my usual tack, though I have to admit I was once left speechless by a boy of no more than eight years old who said, 'Nice tits, missis.' How the hell did *he* know?

'I feel silly'

If you're overweight, or if you're so unfit that your early outings are more walking than running, you may well feel silly. Lots of people are so embarrassed by their early efforts that they run at crack of dawn or dead of night. Even in midsummer, many women run in tracksuit bottoms rather than show their legs. That's why it makes sense to meet other women who've been in the same boat and conquered those feelings. After a while, you'll look snootily down your nose at the non-exercisers and think how silly *they* look.

'It's too hot/cold/wet'

The good old British weather can always be relied upon to be doing the wrong thing. In fact, there's only one weather condition which you shouldn't brave – and that's fog. Its water droplets can irritate the lungs. Besides which, there's always the risk that you'll bump into a lamp-post or, worse, cause a motor accident.

But in all other conditions – there's no excuse! All you need is your most vital resource – common sense.

In hot weather:

★ run in the morning or evening, not in the middle of the day. For town runners this means less pollution as well as a cooler run. If you are on holiday in a hot climate why not run along the beach in the early morning?

★ drink as much water as you can before you go out, and on a long run make sure you can take drinks on the way round.

★ wear light-coloured vest and shorts, preferably made of a material which will allow sweat to evaporate from the skin (see page 145).

In cold and wet weather:

I *love* running in winter. I love coming in after a run in a biting January gale, feeling warm as toast, rosy cheeked and irritatingly self-righteous, then luxuriating in a hot bath and afterwards slurping a steaming bowl of soup. Or running early on Christmas morning before tucking into the turkey. Some people become very low in winter, not to mention putting on a few pounds, and running can shake off all the winter blues. So don't hang up your shoes when the first autumn leaf falls – there's a whole new world out there in the cold and wet, even the snow.

★ You need to be dressed for winter running (see page 146). You'll see some men training in winter in only singlet and shorts. They think it's tough to appear hardy. It isn't. They may be faster than you, but that doesn't make them more sensible.

★ Don't move too far from base, because if you slow down, you can cool very quickly. If you begin to feel slightly dizzy or 'tipsy' stop running, try to find somewhere warm, and then arrange a lift home. Enjoying winter running is one thing – braving the elements in a foolhardy way is quite another.

★ After a winter run, don't hang around in damp clothes. If you can't bath or shower immediately, at least change into dry gear as soon as you can.

★ Drink something warm, like a bowl of porridge, some soup or a mug of cocoa as soon after your run as you can.

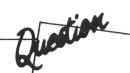

PROJECT 2
WHAT'S STOPPING ME?

For Project 2, I want you to sit down with your husband, and the children (or if you are not married with the person you share your life with) and iron out any potential domestic problems before they occur. Choose a time when you are all relaxed. In your Book, ask your man to write down all the possible reasons he can think of for you not to run. Then go over them with him, item by item.

If your man is a runner, he will probably be very sympathetic and you will be able to count on his support. If he is not, then perhaps you should think about persuading him to start running with you. If he asks questions like 'Who's going to make the dinner/iron my shirts/wash up?' you must have a long discussion about who does what in the house. If you're doing all these things, is it actually fair? Aren't there some domestic tasks he should be sharing, if he doesn't already? Does he spend hours in the pub with his mates while you're stuck with the children at home? Work out between you how you're going to fit running into your lives. Try to answer all the questions he has written in the Book. Tread carefully here, for the idea of this Project is to clear up doubts — not to start a fight!

PROJECT 2
WHAT'S STOPPING ME?

I'm Sue's husband, Jack. Sue has two legs and two arms and there isn't any reason, really, why she shouldn't run, as long as everything gets done around the house.

I suppose I could help a bit, but I'm so knackered when I get in in the evening I like her to look after me.

I *don't* want her going out after dark on her own.

But will she stick to it? Or will it be another seven-day wonder? I'm not sure. She's started so many other things and not carried on with them.

Back to Sue.
Jack basically doesn't believe I can do it — so he doesn't think there are any problems. I'll show him!

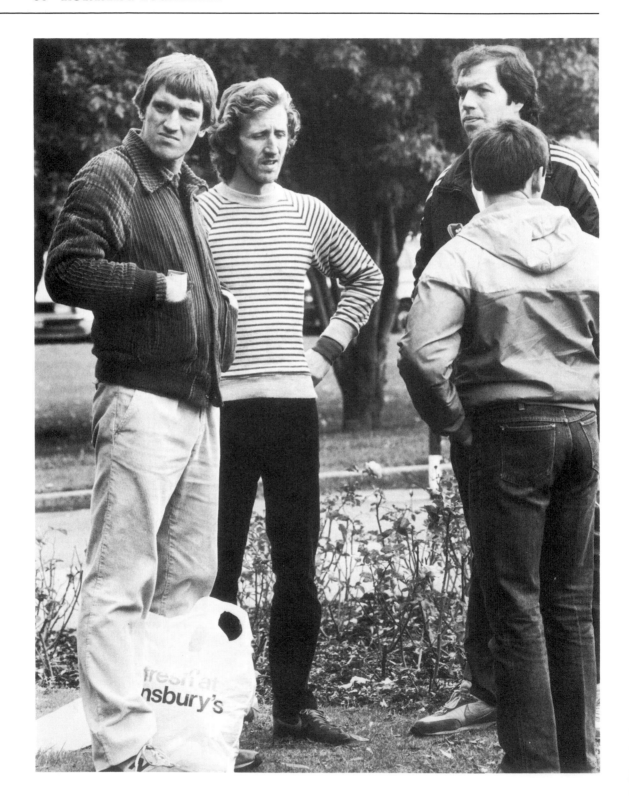

What about the kids?

When Mum starts to run, changes usually have to be made to family life. If your children are old enough, they can run with you and will probably enjoy doing so. Don't take the youngsters too far, though. Children must build up their fitness through a wide range of exercise, and long-distance running is not suitable for those whose bones haven't finished growing. For children aged 4–10 don't go further than about three miles; for children aged 11–16 no further than seven; 16–18 no further than 14.

If your children are tiny, you will need to find someone to look after them. If your husband, childminder, or older children cannot help, your best plan is to form a group with other mothers and take it in turns to mind the children. Or do as Wendy Surawy and her friends did when they first started running. In the absence of babyminders, they pushed the children in their buggies round Streatham Common. The children loved it!

'What about my husband or boyfriend?'

What about him? What does he think about your ambition to start running regularly? Though the decision is yours alone, you need to be taken seriously, and you will need his co-operation.

Changes will occur in your family and the Man-in-your-life may have to adapt, too.

CHAPTER THREE
Running together

Some of us are 'loners' — preferring to run alone, free, in our own time, at our own pace. We think of this solo running as 'breathing space', 'thinking time', 'escape valve' or 'holiday' and treasure the time away from the screaming children or the telephone. That's fine. But for every 'loner' there are a dozen women who don't want to run alone — either because they are afraid, or because they just cannot make any progress without someone else to encourage them. If you're one of these women, what you need is a 'Sister'. Let me tell you how the Sisters Project started, and what it is.

Women have been slow to catch on to the jogging and running boom. The boom, which came to Britain from the USA, revolved round the marathon – 26 miles, 385 yards – which it appears women were reluctant to tackle – for in the first London Marathon only eight per cent of the field were women, and in other marathons around the country, the percentage was never more than about 10 per cent.

Market research carried for *Running* magazine at the beginning of 1983 suggested that only eight per cent of readers were women. *Running*'s Editor, Andy Etchells, columnist Geoffrey Cannon and I spent some weeks hatching a scheme to encourage more women to run, and to read the magazine.

It was easy to see *why* there weren't so many women running – they were afraid to go out alone, but couldn't join a club – either because they were afraid they'd be too slow to join a club, or because they couldn't manage the regular evening meetings because of family or work responsibilities.

I had some *awful* early experiences when I started running that I wouldn't wish on other women. I'd go along to find a group of people (mostly men) warming up and doing exotic-looking stretching exercises, and then there'd be a 'pip-pip' of digital watches and

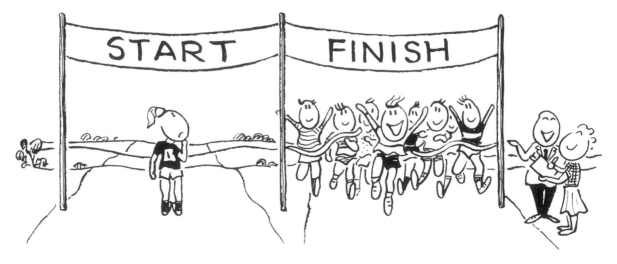

the people would all vanish over the horizon, leaving me for dead. Another time, I went along hoping to cover four miles for the first time. I was put into the wrong group and ended up doing four miles for the first *and* second times – together! When I arrived back from my unintended eight-miler, I discovered that my tracksuit was locked away in a car and the owner was running 18 miles and I had to shiver till he came back . . . I knew that other women had had these ghastly experiences too, and that many had been put off running as a result.

People love writing to magazines, and there is nothing like being a 'guinea pig' for making them stick to training schedules. The previous year, 1982, we had launched the Fun Runner 82 project in which we trained 34 everyday unfit London folk (men and women) to run *The Sunday Times* Fun Run. Not only had these people become fit and streamlined – they had also become very enthusiastic about the way running had changed their lives for the better.

We wanted to launch another project like Fun Runner 82 but particularly geared to women. We would look at the lifestyles, attitudes and health of women taking up running for the first time and compare them with women who were already running.

It was to be a straightforward research project – with a 'control' group of runners and a 'experimental' group of non-runners – until I threw a spanner in the works with the most unscientific suggestion that instead of looking at the two groups separately we paired the women up – runner with non-runner, so that the experienced women could help the beginners through their first few steps.

We would set the beginners (we called them Little Sisters) a target – the all-women Avon Cosmetics 10-mile race to be held in October of that particular year – and persuade the runners (Big Sisters) to cajole, encourage, advise and sympathise throughout the five-month training period. We would publish monthly schedules in the magazine aimed at runners of all standards. And we would supply the runners with diary pages to fill in and return to us so that we could write about their progress in the magazine.

If I'd known what I was letting myself in for, I would have given up there and then. I couldn't have foreseen that within 18 months my simple idea would have persuaded more than 4,000 women to start running.

Andy Etchells agreed to a small announcement in the back of *Running*, which we figured no-one would read anyway, because it was a specialist magazine read mostly by men. How wrong we were! Those men passed the announcement on to wives and girlfriends, secretaries and bosses – or in some cases wrote the letters themselves on behalf of women who were too shy to reply! We were deluged with mail – there were days when the caretaker was barely visible under stacks of envelopes marked 'Sisters Project'.

Margaret Johnstone, 36, from St Albans, wrote: 'Husband pointed out invitation in magazine. Tried to ignore it. Thought of winter flab I'd like to lose . . .

'Re-read. Remembered cheering husband in Burnham half-marathon, Luton 10. Looked at lovely slim women, with visions of being among them. Back to jogging round the block.

'Look at 11-year-old daughter out training with Dad. Decide to stick to music teaching. Make excuses not to go jogging.

An invitation...

We at **Running Magazine** want to see more women running in 1983. But getting started isn't always easy. Now's your big chance to start running – if you're a beginner – or, if you're already a regular runner, to pass the word and the enjoyment on by getting someone else started.

This time last year I issued an invitation to beginners to form a group with the goal of completing the *Sunday Times* National Fun Run. Fun Runner '82 was formed, with 64 participants, although I received over 130 applications, with women in the majority.

This year my invitation is to women only, and the aim is higher. I'm looking for women who are willing to train for the Avon 10 mile race to be held at Copthall Stadium, Hendon, north London, on Sunday October 2 – the biggest women's only event on the British running calendar. The first event in 1981 attracted 153 women, the second 276. This year, even if you've never run before, you could be there too!

I'm looking for two groups of women. First, absolute beginners. It's all right if you jog a bit, but the more unfit you are, the better. If the idea of completing a 10-mile race six months from now seems ridiculous, better still. Second, runners. To qualify as a runner you should already have run a 10-mile race (or half-marathon or marathon). It doesn't matter how fast or slow you are, as long as you have the experience of running 10 miles and are currently in regular training.

We'll pair each beginner off, one-to-one with a "big sister" – a woman from the runners' group matched as far as possible for geographical region, age group and lifestyle. The "sisters" will keep in regular touch with each other – the runners imparting advice, enthusiasm and assurance to the beginners. In addition **Running Magazine** will publish a regular training schedule and progress reports between now and October in my *Fun Runner* column.

This is your opportunity to join. Please write by April 22 for an application form to me, Geoffrey Cannon, at **Running**, 57-61 Mortimer St, London W1 7TD. Mark your envelope Sisters Project and enclose a large stamped addressed envelope.

In your letter please also state whether you are a beginner or a runner (with details of your running/racing background), and give your age, weight, height, occupation and address. It doesn't matter where you live as long as you are prepared to come to London under your own steam (and at your own expense!) to run the Avon 10 on October 2.

The training programme will start on May 1, which allows everyone five months. For the moment, just believe that this will be enough time!

'Look at *Running* magazine again. Ten miles is out of the question. Panic! What if I come last? Avon 10 is for athletes, which I'm not at 4ft 10½in without shoes and 9½st (ugh). Throw magazine in dustbin.

'Jog a couple of miles. Feel better. Retrieve magazine. Where's the page? Help!!'

Jackie Keen, 35, wrote from Colchester: 'For some time now I have been desperate for the inspiration to get fit and lose weight – your programme seems custom built! I can't run 200 yards without stopping for a rest. The Avon 10 may be just the target I need.'

'I *desperately* need the spur!' said Marion Leslie, 39, of London.

The balance of experienced runners to beginners came out almost exactly 1–2, so we gave each Big Sister two Little Sisters. This threesome idea worked out very well, because even if one woman dropped out, the other two could keep going, and two Little Sisters could run together.

The most important single benefit of the Sisters Project is that women found new friends – friends from different ages and lifestyles. Some of these friendships extended beyond just running together – Carol Charlesworth of Pinner now sees more of her little sisters Judy and Liz socially than she does to run.

Many of the friendships cut across age groups and differences in occupations and lifestyle. Big Sister Val Collinson was delighted to go for post-run breakfasts at her Little Sister's house. 'They've got an Aga!' she told me enthusiastically.

Women also found that they could share skills and resources outside running – from caring for each other's children to financial, medical or legal help. For some the Project was a real eye-opener. Childless women gained more understanding of how a busy mother has to make elaborate plans and timetables to enable her to fit in a training run while 'household mums' escaped from the house to meet other women of all ages and occupations.

For some women the Project didn't work because their Sisters were just too far away – though that didn't stop Linda Reed of Warminster becoming firm friends with Robbie Spooner in Sherborne, some 24 miles as the crow flies. Irene Ashton, Shan Trow and Frances Classon all live in Clwyd, but it's a big county, and Holywell, Ruthin and Wrexham aren't exactly near neighbours. This didn't stop them meeting to run and exchange tips and advice.

One reason I feel the Sisters Project worked is that women are naturally more caring and sharing than men – a woman who runs faster than you isn't going to go haring off and leave you behind. It can be very demoralising to see the apparent ease with which an overweight and unfit man can turn in a better performance. It is much easier for a woman to find the support and encouragement she needs when taking those first steps if she is running with other women who understand the sort of problems she is likely to have.

Many women who volunteered as Big Sisters thought we wouldn't want them because they were slow, or hadn't been running for very long. And yet these turned out to be ideal qualifications for a Big Sister. Some of the best and most appreciated Big Sisters were those who had their early running days fresh in their memories and who didn't run that much faster than their charges (in some cases, a good deal *slower!*).

Half way through the Project, Diana Scott wrote from Yorkshire of the 'embarrassing fact that the Little Sisters have suddenly started to look big! From 12-minute miles I am now doing 10-minute miles quite easily, and my Sisters (Ann Leach and Anne Craven) are pushing *me* into single figures. I don't know what I've done, but *they're* marvellous!' A clear case of the boot on the other foot.

It was possible for a Big Sister to train a beginner and improve herself. Some Big Sisters needed the motivation as much as the beginners. 'I had just gone through a bad patch after my first and only marathon,' said Corinne Roberts from Bradford, 'but the Project gave me a reason to go on.' Maureen Farish and her training partner Nanette Cross from Bromley had just completed the London Marathon. 'Where do we go now?' they wondered. 'With the Sisters Project we were given a new and seemingly insurmountable goal to reach.' These women took pride and pleasure in the achievements of the beginners under their wing. Some Big Sisters found that they were so busy worrying about their Little Sisters that they forgot their own problems!

Three's company

Although the women started off in groups of three, many found that their groups grew until they had gained an entirely new social circle. Running gently within their limitations, they could talk on the run. 'We discuss everything,' says Maria Williams of Harlow, 'from running to the price of bacon.' Big Sister Brenda Green from Enfield now has over 80 women under her wing, and delights in the changes that running has brought about in them. 'They come to me for help,' she says, 'overweight, overtired and over the hill. But after a few months of gentle jogging the signs of improvement are there – glowing skins, sparkling eyes, a trimmer shape, and that look of confidence and well-being.'

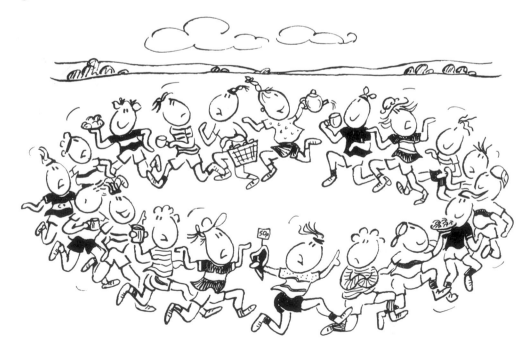

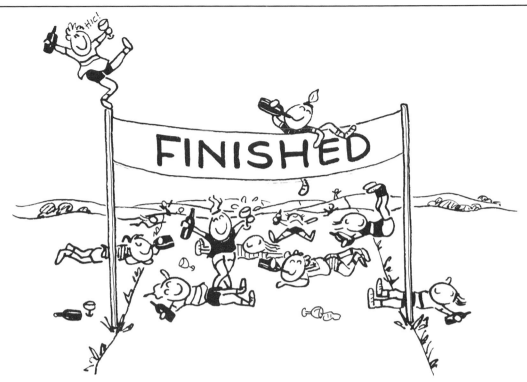

Clubbing together

Many Big Sisters were members of athletic or jogging clubs in their area – clubs that the Little Sisters would be frightened of joining for fear that they weren't good enough. The Big Sisters were able to judge for themselves when it would be right to introduce their Little Sisters to club life. Then the beginners could meet others of the same standard and be reassured that the club was the right place for them. With this confidence they improved by leaps and bounds, as well as making many new friends. And one of the biggest benefits was that of safety in numbers. 'We all feel a lot safer, and our husbands are much more content to let us go running after dark,' says Maria Williams.

Big Sisters also gently introduced their charges to races. Viv Williamson of Colindale took her Little Sisters Sue Carter and Ann Boxshall to a five-mile race before the Avon 10. 'I'd hate to be responsible for them arriving at the Avon 10 all green and untried,' she said. 'Bottles of expensive wine changed hands in the form of bribes for any time under 50 minutes. It was a very expensive day for me.'

Contagious enthusiasm

Many of the Sisters found that their enthusiasm was contagious and that friends and workmates soon took a lively interest in their progress. Some women felt that running improved their relationships with male colleagues, and they found they could communicate on a more equal footing than some of their non-sporting friends.

At home, the Sisters valued the support of their families. Many husbands and boyfriends took up running for the first time, while those women who regarded themselves as 'running widows' had a new insight into why running played such an important part in their man's life.

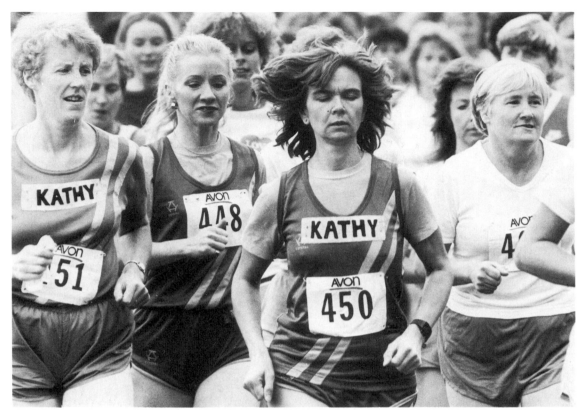

448 Jill Jackson and 450 Kathleen Moody are members of their company's running club, Peak Freans AC.

2 October 1983

In a record British field of 881 runners, 150 Little Sisters, who had only started training on 1 May, finished the Avon Cosmetics National 10-mile road racing championships. It sounds grand. It *was* grand. Husbands, boyfriends, children, pals turned out in force to support the women – even Sisters who, frustratingly, couldn't run the race themselves because they were ill or injured.

Were those supporters impressed? You bet. The doubting Thomases were struck dumb, while other men, whose wives had doubted their own ability, said, smugly, 'I knew she could.'

I've given the race times here to give you some idea of the standard I'm talking about – the winner of that race, Angela Tooby, completed the course in 55½ minutes. There is pride in every achievement, however slow.

'Mine must be the proudest family in Woking' (Jenny Westall, 1:52)

'They didn't really think I'd stick it out – they are proud of me' (Joan Seamer, 1:34)

'"HELLO, CHAMP" said my husband, James. "I knew you could do it!"' (Betty Mackinnon, 1:59)

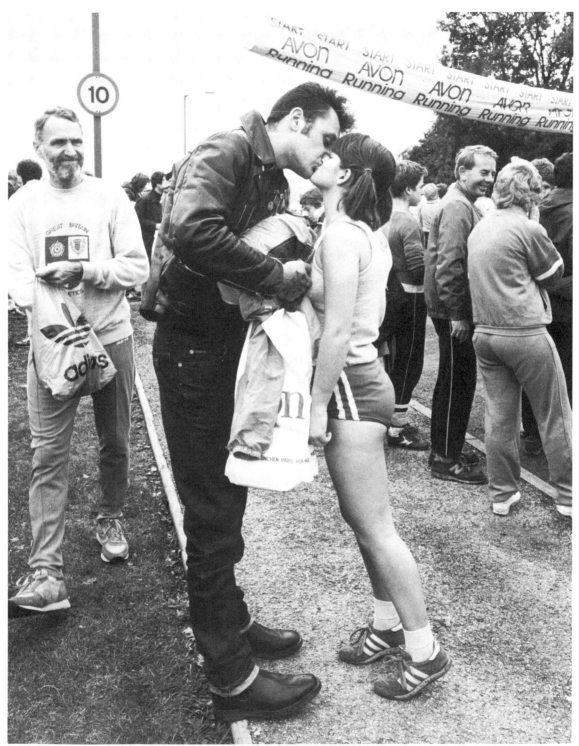

'It was the first time he'd told me he was proud of me.'

'Mike came and took photos. He said I was going "like a tank" – so he wasn't surprised I finished' (Pam Davison, 1:22)

'Steve is really proud of me and my mum and gran phoned to congratulate me. They're all really pleased' (Moira Chilton, 1:32)

'Gill has called me the "slave driver" but really, I have never needed to be. Just look at her – 48 years old, mother of five (oldest 24, youngest 10). She has stuck to the schedule like a limpet. If she takes on something she'll see it through, believe me. I'm as proud of her as can be' (Gordon Nicholas of his wife, Gill, 1:35)

'The praise from my husband has been non-stop' (Irene Allen, 1:47)

Euphoria
The race finished inside the stadium with a band playing and all the supporters cheering from the grandstand. For many women (including me) it was a very emotional occasion.

'I had a lump in my throat when the gun went off, and an even bigger lump when I heard the band playing at the finish' (Karen Schofield, 1:41)

'What an atmosphere! On entering the stadium at the finish I felt like an Olympic Marathon runner on the home straight!' (Barbara Lowe, 1:32)

'I felt euphoric – after a good run the previous weekend I decided to give the whole 10 miles a go – and did not expect to maintain the pace' (Liz Bardsley, 1:39)

'I didn't finish last!' (Jean Thomas, 1:27)

'To cap a great day I met Joyce Smith after the race, who congratulated me and encouraged me to keep on with my running. I walked away on air!' (Diane Dean, 1:24)

'YIPPEE!' (Joy Siegel, 1:39)

Well done, Sister
Many women paid tribute to their Sisters' achievement, and the role they played in their own success.

'I couldn't have done it without Maria. To stop now would be terrible – so the first thing we did was make arrangements for our next run' (Pat Ashford, 1:33)

'I would never have done it without Pat' (Maria Williams, 1:33). (Maria and Pat were neighbouring Little Sisters who did all their training together)

'Jean and Pam were tremendous. I saw them before the start, terribly nervous and aiming for something around 90–100 minutes. So what did they do? Jean, from a base of nothing did 87 minutes and Pam, from a little jogging, did 82! I was so pleased for them both' (Big Sister Kay Gillespie, 1:09, of her Little Sisters Jean Thomas and Pam Davison)

A kick up the backside
After the race, Karen Schofield from Bracknell wrote: 'The Sisters Project has been my

kick up the backside. It has given me goals, guidance, schedules, encouragement, running mates and inspiration.'

The Project was the push that the beginners needed to get themselves out of the front door and the encouragement that they needed to keep going – encouragement they hadn't found in other ways of keeping fit. It was also a vital boost for those women who had started to run but hadn't been able to keep it up regularly.

'The Sisters Project helped enormously to get me off the ground,' wrote Inger Baud of Churchdown. 'I had tried to run on a regular basis many times before, but I never managed more than two or three miles about three times a week. With the Project I had the encouragement to do it properly and gradually build up more miles, whereas before I didn't have the confidence to go further.'

An important feature of the Project was the detailed training diary which every Sister was asked to complete and send off to *Running* every four or five weeks. The fear of submitting blank pages was another incentive to stick to the training and diary keeping.

Inger Baud again: 'Filling in the Diary on a daily basis made a great difference. It was nice to share my ups and downs with somebody.' We'll be looking at these ups and down in more detail, and finding out just how important it is to keep a diary in a later chapter.

Throughout the Project, Lesley Dean of Evesham told herself, 'Look, I have to do this, because I'm in the Sisters Project and I can't let them down.' Lynne Butler, from Woodford Green, told everyone what she was doing – that way it made it more difficult to backslide – and Pauline Hopkins of Birmingham 'felt a part of something very important. I proved to myself and others that the most ordinary of women were capable of completing a physical programme.'

PROJECT 3
FIND A RUNNING MATE

If you want to start running and reaping the benefits that these women have done, then, like them, you need some motivation and encouragement. So the next thing you need to do is find a running mate.

Think of all the people you know. There must be someone (woman *or* man) at work, in your road, in your family, in your dance class, at the school gates, who would like to start running with you.

Pluck up the courage to ask. The Projects in the next few chapters will become tougher, and you'll be glad of a friend or two as you tackle them.

If you really cannot find anyone to run with, write to me at *Running* magazine, 57–61 Mortimer Street, London W1N 7TD, and I'll put you in touch with a Big Sister in your area. She may even be someone you've already met.

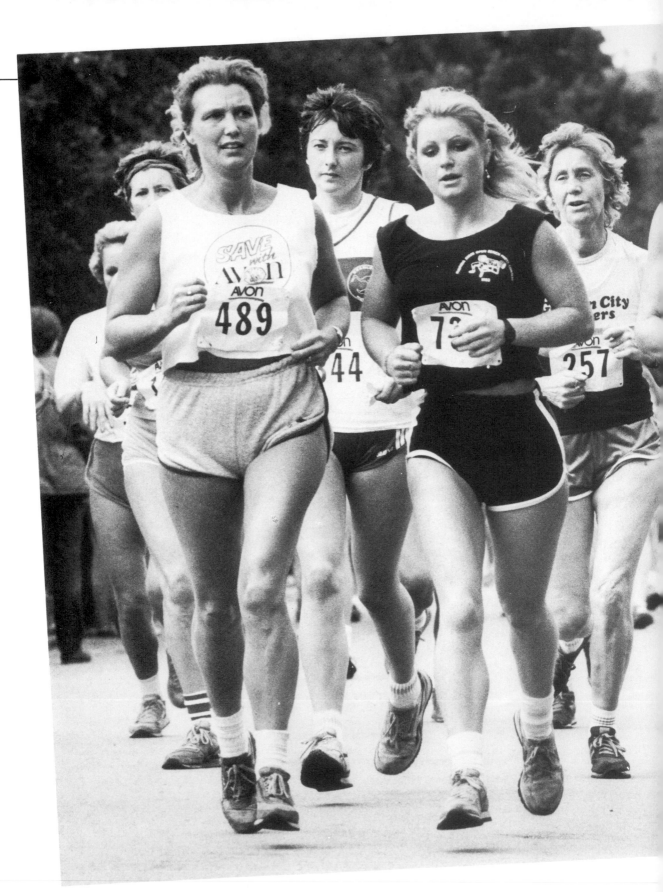

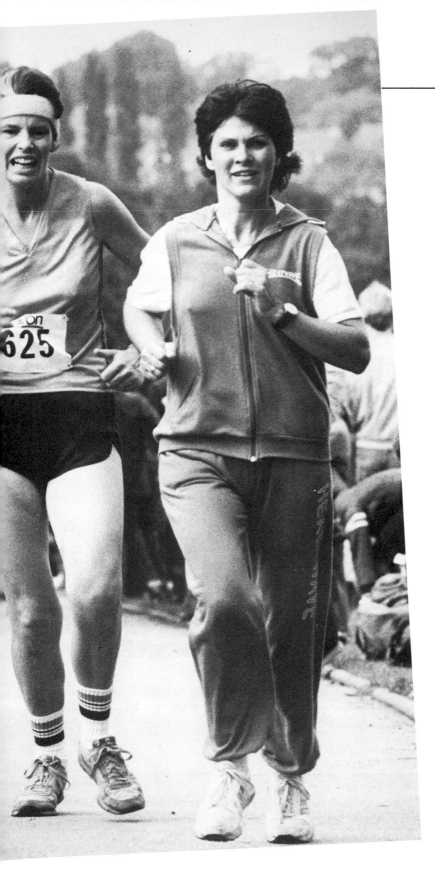

489 Pat Smith looks comfortable, but 625 Rosey Foster doesn't necessarily agree

CHAPTER FOUR
How are you?

'Hello, how are you?' How often do you greet people like this? Every day, I'm sure. But how often do you wait for an answer? Do you care how the other person is? When they say, 'I'm fine, how are you?' or 'OK, but...' are you really interested? I want to know how you are. If you're not feeling 100 per cent, if you belong to the 'OK, but...' brigade you know you could feel better, but you don't know how to *get* better – this book can help you.

The magic potion

You must sometimes wish that there was a magic potion which, at one fell swoop, would:

★ cure your tensions and headaches
★ help you sleep and then help you wake bright-eyed
★ take 10 years off your age
★ whittle away that extra half-stone
★ increase your circle of friends
★ help you give up smoking
★ put colour in your cheeks, a shine in your hair and a spring in your step

Well, there isn't. It's not possible to buy it over a chemist's counter.

Running is the next best thing. It won't change your life overnight, nor will it do all those good things at once. But, as you've already seen, more and more women are finding that running can bring about long-term changes in their lives – changes for the better that they don't want to reverse. Each, in her own way, has found the bottle of magic potion.

Where do you begin?

For the moment, never mind how *fit* you are. Are you *well*? Your body and your common sense will tell you what that means. If you have had flu or a fever, or been sick or had diarrhoea or if you have been coughing fit to burst, you don't need me or a doctor to tell you that you aren't well; that you should rest and wait till you feel better.

With some chronic (long-lasting) illnesses you *can* start running. Do you suffer from any of the following?

★ high blood pressure
★ heart disease or a family history of heart disease
★ asthma
★ diabetes
★ bronchitis
★ back pain

★ you are seriously overweight
★ you smoke more than 20 cigarettes a day
★ anything else which requires regular medicine

The good news is that none of these conditions rules out running; the even better news is that running can *help* you in most cases. But you should keep your doctor informed of your intention to run so that s/he can make adjustments to any medicine you are taking. I'm not counting pregnancy as an illness here, but as a healthy state of body and mind which we'll examine later.

Doctors are strangely divided on the subject of exercise. Regular exercise is the cheapest and most enduring prescription for a long, full life, and it beats me why so many GPs are still so keen to prescribe expensive tranquillisers and sedatives as cures for today's problems. If you are not happy with your doctor's advice, change – find a doctor who speaks your language! Ask her/him if drugs are the only answer to your problems – or can exercise help you?

If you feel well, there's no reason why you shouldn't start to run. First, it's time for you and your running mate to try a simple test to see how fit you are.

Project 4 is a simple *aerobic* exercise. You could be forgiven for thinking that 'aerobics' is a rather energetic form of dancing which involves leaping up and down in front of mirrors, wearing brightly-coloured skin-tight clothes. 'Aerobic' has become a rather general and sometimes misused word to cover the dance and fitness boom – but it means much more.

Any exercise is aerobic if it 'promotes the supply and use of oxygen'. So says Dr Ken Cooper, one of the pioneers of the exercise boom in the USA and the author of several books on the subject. Being aerobically fit means that your lungs can take in more oxygen from the air you breathe. It also means having a strong heart which has to pump fewer times to get that oxygen round the bloodstream – not only for the vital arteries that supply your brain, your muscles and your digestive organs, but every blood vessel, too. A fit body works like a well-oiled machine, efficiently burning up the food you eat and the oxygen you breathe, and eliminating the waste products your body doesn't need.

In touch with your pulse

You may think of your pulse as something the doctor takes when you are ill – though taking your pulse then is a bit meaningless because neither you nor the doctor have anything to compare it with. If your pulse is normally quite high or low, how does the doctor really know how ill you are?

Try to think of your pulse, or heart rate, as a measure of good health, not illness. If you take your pulse regularly, daily or weekly, you will be able to see how your fitness is improving.

Your *resting pulse* is your heart rate when you wake in the morning, or when you are so relaxed in the evening that you are unable to move out of the armchair to go to bed! You have about six pints of blood in your body, and at rest this makes about one circuit per minute of the body, from the heart, out through the arteries to your brain, the muscles of your arms and legs, and your digestive organs. As you become fitter your resting heart rate goes down.

Question

PROJECT 4
THE SKIPPING TEST

Time to get out of the armchair — this is an *active* Project! You'll need:

★ your Book
★ a pen or pencil
★ any watch or clock (with hands *or* digits) that shows the seconds clearly
★ a skipping rope — buy a proper one with handles, or simple use a suitable length of sash cord or washing line from your local hardware store.

This is a test that you can do indoors, preferably on soft carpet in bare or stockinged feet. Don't do the test, or indeed any exercise, within two hours of a meal, a cigarette, or an alcoholic drink.

I want you to skip, on alternate feet, for 250 skips. Don't worry if you stumble or trip, just get going again smoothly as soon as you can. Don't rush, but keep skipping steadily. Try not to stop, unless you really feel awful, before the 250 skips are completed.

Now sit down and relax, making sure that you've got your Book and pen handy.

How do you feel? Put your hand on your heart. Feel it beating. Don't count the beats just yet, we'll do that a bit later on. Listen to your breathing. Are you gasping for breath or breathing comfortably? Look at your face in the mirror? Is it red? Or moist? Do you have any pain in the chest? Do you feel dizzy, or lightheaded? Spend some time writing down how you feel, and the changes that are going on in your body as you gradually recover from your first exertion. How long does it take before you feel your body is back to normal? Some of you will feel awful and ready to give up here and now. Well, things can only improve, I can assure you.

Answer

PROJECT 4
HOW ARE YOU?

250 skips – completed with a few trips. Otherwise OK.

You're joking! I'm *shattered*! My heart feels as if its bursting out of my chest. I'm red faced, hot and sticky. It doesn't *hurt*, exactly, and I don't feel dizzy.

2 minutes later: my heart has slowed down a bit. I'm *yawning*. I don't want to get out of the chair yet but I do feel a bit better.

5 minutes later. I'm going to get up and make a cup of tea now. My heart is still beating quite fast. My face isn't so red.

10 minutes later: I feel dozy. I'm still yawning! But everything else seems to be back to normal.

500 skips and pulse counting.

I somehow managed to start more slowly, so it wasn't such a shock to my system!

Pulse before exercise. 20 beats in 15 seconds = 80 beats a minute.

Immediately after	$40 \times 4 = 160$
Two mins after	$37 \times 4 = 148$
Five mins after	$35 \times 4 = 140$
10 mins after	$24 \times 4 = 96$

Mmm. It didn't take *too* long to get back to normal, I suppose. Same effect as last time. I wanted to drop off to sleep!

Taking your pulse
Some people can barely find a pulse in their wrists, where the doctor usually takes it, and feel a stronger beat on the side of the neck alongside the major artery linking the heart and the brain, the body's equivalent of the M1 motorway.

Always take your resting pulse in the same way, and at the same time of day. The best time is first thing in the morning. Using your watch, count the number of beats in 15 seconds and then multiply by four to give you the number of beats per minute. You may want to find someone else to do the timing for you. Practice makes perfect, so don't worry if your measurements jump up and down the first few times. When you're happy with your resting pulse measurements, you are ready to try taking your pulse *after* exercise.

Maximum heart rate

When you exercise, instead of a leisurely one lap of the body, your blood goes round much faster, up to five laps in a minute. There is a safe limit, though, to the work you can expect your heart to do. In your early days as a runner, you probably won't reach this limit before your body asks you to stop. Later on, though, you'll be able to push yourself a little closer to this limit which, as a rough guide, is 200 beats a minute for people up to 20 years of age, then 220 (minus your age in years) after that.

Recovery time

The last important thing you need to know about your heart is the amount of time it takes to recover after exercise. When you finished skipping, how long did that exhausted feeling last? One minute, five minutes, an hour, or were you whacked for the rest of the day? The fitter you become, the sooner you will be able to recover from your exertions.

When you first start to run, you will probably feel too tired to do anything afterwards, and you may start to worry that running is taking up too much of your energy and that you won't be able to stay awake at your desk or lift the Hoover. Don't worry! In a few weeks, the tide will have turned. You'll run back through your front door feeling tired all right, but after a soak in the bath, or a shower, and a reviving drink you'll be ready for anything!

Now I want you do the same skipping test again. This time take your pulse before and after the test, timing the test, and recording how long it takes you to recover.

Sitting comfortably, take your 'before' pulse. This may not be as 'rested' as your early morning pulse if you've been up a few hours, so don't worry. Count the number of beats in 15 seconds and multiply by four. Write down this figure.

Now skip 500 times, not rushing, but steadily. Don't worry how long it takes, but try not to stop. When you have finished, sit down and take your pulse. Write the figure down again. Two minutes after finishing, take your pulse again; then again at five and 10 minutes after finishing. Then, as you did before, write down any other feelings you have about the test.

In touch with yourself

You may never have taken your own pulse before. How does it feel to be in touch with your body and understand how a part of it, the most important part, works? Measuring your aerobic fitness regularly is many times more important than jumping on and off the scales to measure the tiniest weight loss.

There are more elaborate tests you can do (or have done) to measure your fitness, but they are tests which set you up against the 'norms' of other people. You can pay £25 or more to be told that, for a woman of 38 years and 11st 3lb, you are in 'poor', 'average' or 'fair' shape, and then later on shell out again to be told that you are now 'good', 'very good' or 'excellent' for a woman of your age and weight.

I want *you* to be the judge of your own fitness. Many times as we go through the book and its Projects I'll urge you to 'listen' to your body, to write down what it tells you, and to keep a careful diary so that you'll come to know *exactly* how you are.

CHAPTER FIVE
Finding your feet

When you're servicing a car, you don't just look under the bonnet at
the engine – you look at the chassis, too. You make sure the wheels
are balanced and turning smoothly, and you make sure the tyres
have some tread in them and that they are inflated to the right
pressure. For however much you have spent on the latest in turbo-
charging, fuel injection and other modern marvels, it's wasted if the
bodywork isn't up to scratch.

In Chapter Four, we only looked under the bonnet at ways of making your body's engine
run more smoothly. Now it's time to oil the wheels, pump up the tyres and get moving.
Just as you have become a little more aware of how your heart and lungs work, I want
you to spend some time finding out about your legs and feet.

When Upright Man came down from the trees over a million years ago, he began to
streamline his body for hunting and fishing. Today's model, *homo sapiens*, appears to
have ironed out many of the design faults of the earlier models, and runs rather
smoothly. Upright Woman, on the other hand, seems to have kept many of those design
faults as standard features. Only a few lucky women can be described as graceful
runners. The rest of us find, when we run, that our hips and breasts stick out and our
bottoms wobble. When we are pregnant, our spines sag under the weight and our feet
turn inwards. Looking ungraceful may be one of the things that holds you back.

But let's think on the bright side. This book is about making the best of what you
have, whether you're built like a Ferrari or a Morris Minor, a racehorse or a Thelwell
pony.

I expect some of you are becoming a little impatient with me. 'What's the point of
Project 5?' you're probably saying. 'I've been walking since . . . well, since I could
walk.' Exactly. Walking is such a natural activity that you just do it without thinking
about it. And if you're not thinking about it, it's easy to develop bad habits. When you
walk just a short way each day these bad habits don't matter, but when you start to run
regularly, you can run into problems!!

In running a mile, each foot will be hitting the ground at least 800 times. You're
attached to that foot, all eight, nine, 10 or more stone of you. For a 10-stoner that's
about 250 tons per foot, per mile. If you have a bad habit when you're walking it's going
to show itself up many more times when you're running. That, simply, is how many new
runners become injured. But I want to keep you off the physio's couch and out of the
doctor's surgery, so it's best to iron out all your design faults before you take to the road.

Walk around the room again. Are you knock-kneed? Bow-legged? Pigeon-toed?
Flat-footed? Again, try and concentrate on a rhythmic heel-toe stride with both feet
facing straight forward. Make more notes in your Book. It's not true that you can't teach
an old dog new tricks. You *can* change the way you walk and run – for the better. When
Janet Bowden of Bromley started running, she admits she had 'several weeks of assorted
joint problems with a lot of pain – before realising I *could* adjust and re-train my "style"
to overcome these problems'.

Question

PROJECT 5
WALKABOUT

Before you start running properly, it's time for a test drive. Project 5, you'll be pleased to hear, is nothing like as strenuous as the skipping test. This time I want you to move slowly and thoughtfully, paying special attention to your hips, legs, and feet. For this project you'll need:

★ outdoor clothes
★ your front door key
★ any flat shoes
★ a mission – a shopping trip, a walk to the station, a letter to post, or someone to visit. This should be about 10–15 minutes away. It doesn't matter if you also have a pram to push, or something heavy to carry.
★ your Book and pen ready for when you return.

Off you go, just walking steadily. Don't shuffle, but walk with a rhythmic heel-toe action. If your feet naturally turn inwards or outwards, try and make them face straight ahead. Think about what is happening in your legs and feet as you move forwards. Think about the movement of the joints between your bones.

★ Are your joints flexible and free-moving, or are they stiff?
★ Do your muscles feel elastic or tight?
★ Is one leg stronger than the other?
★ Do your strides seem even?
★ Are you limping, or shifting your weight unevenly from side to side?
★ Are your shoulders and hips swinging too much from side to side?
★ Are you in any pain?

Back indoors, kick your shoes off and walk around barefoot for a while. Then sit down and relax and write your reactions in your Book.

High heels — the worst habit of all

One of the commonest problems faced by women running for the first time is pain in the area of the Achilles tendon.

The muscles in this region become shortened if you wear high heels regularly, and stretching them out in a natural running action can hurt for the first few times until you're used to it. In Chapter Six I'll show you a gentle stretching exercise which will make the transition easier.

Other things happen to your feet if you wear fashion shoes all the time. To understand them, try doing Project 5 – Walkabout – again in your favourite heeled shoes. Ouch! How far did you get? Write down the differences you notice.

★ Are your toes cramped into the front of the shoe at every stride?
★ Do your heels wobble about as they (or the shoes) come into contact with the ground?
★ Or look at other women as you walk behind them in the street. Note how awkward *their* feet look crammed into ill-fitting shoes.

Walk tall

I've been 5ft 9in since I was 11, so I'm not really the person to liberate you from uncomfortable shoes if you barely stand 4ft 9in. Neither is the Princess of Wales, who started the present trend towards sensible 'flatties' – she's 5ft 10in, and though she sometimes wears high heels they bring her well above her husband.

It's worth remembering that there are many successful small men around who don't totter about in silly shoes. My teenage heartthrob was Dudley Moore, all 5ft 3in of him. His height, or lack of it, has been a positive asset because he developed a talent and personality that made people look up to him. And he's not the only example of a small man who's been successful.

PROJECT 5
WALKABOUT

I walked the children to school, with Matthew in the buggy. I do it every day, and it was funny trying to break down the movements into small parts. Easier coming back without distraction from the older children.

My legs certainly seem to be a disaster area! I felt like an old woman – very stiff. I shuffle and scuff along, without really moving my joints at all. Yes, they are stiff. My right leg seems stronger – makes a bigger stride. My hips are all over the place.

Does it hurt? No, but now I'm thinking about them my legs feel very tired. My feet turn inwards a little bit – I hadn't noticed that before.

In the afternoon, I tried walking to school with my heels on. It *did* feel odd, and wobbly. I walked behind Carl's mother and noticed how her legs were moving. She was wearing high heeled sandals. She looked a bit wobbly, too.

I was glad to get those shoes off when I got in. I usually am. I didn't realise it was because I am forcing my feet down inside them. Perhaps I'll stick with the 'flatties'.

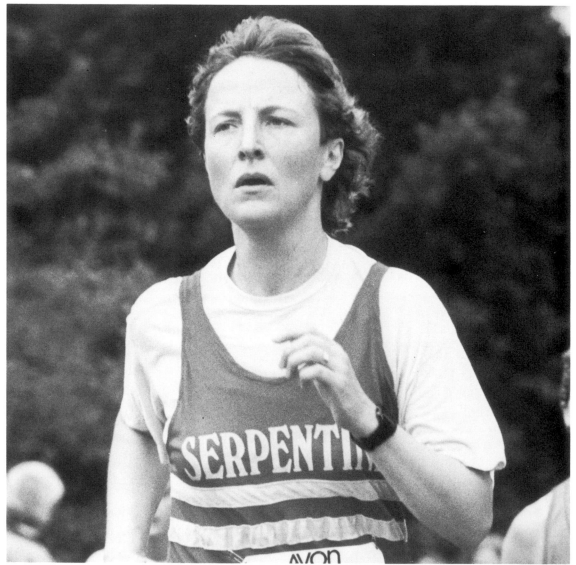

Dumpy daughter turned runner, author Alison Turnbull

The only person who can make you stand tall without high heels is *you*. As you become fitter, more flexible and more self-confident, you may just find you don't need them any more – however tall or short you are. Always think about walking tall, and you'll run tall, too.

Compared with other sports, running is a very cheap and versatile hobby. You don't need lessons, a court, a racket, a boat or a roof rack. You don't need to travel miles to find a calm sea and a following wind; and you don't need to call up 10 other people to make sure they can all turn up on Saturday afternoon. Just pull on your gear, step out of the front door, and you're off . . . in theory.

The right shoes

But what gear? Don't worry about clothing for the moment. Take Judy Wurr's advice: 'Shoes are of the utmost importance. Forget the trendy headbands, sun visors, pink tracksuits, matching earrings . . .'

The most important thing to do now, before you start running, is to buy a good pair of running *shoes*. Don't assume that any old tennis shoes, plimsolls or other flat shoes will 'do'. Just as you can't eat soup with a fork, or slice bread with a spoon, you need specialised shoes for your chosen sport. For tennis and squash you need shoes that will support your feet through sideways and twisting movements, while for running you need shoes that will support your feet in forward movement and absorb the shock of each footfall.

Gimmicks apart, the two most important things to look for in a running shoe are the *midsole* and the *heel counter*. The midsole is an extra layer of (usually white) shock-absorbent material which cushions your foot as you run over cracks, rocks, cobbles and bumps. The heel counter is a cup made either of plastic or reinforced board which wraps around the back of the shoe and stops your heel moving from side to side each time your foot hits the ground.

SHOE BUYING TIPS

Take your time. When you go to a running shop, be prepared to spend some time there – don't nip in and out with your purchase in five minutes. Avoid the type of shop where the shoes are proudly displayed on shoe trees or stuffed with newspaper. They're not greeengrocery – you should be able to pick them up, feel inside them, bend them, examine them, and, most important, try them on.

PROJECT 6
BUYING YOUR SHOES

It's worth phoning a few shops in your area before making the trek to buy your shoes. Ask for recommendations for a woman just starting out. A good retailer keeps abreast of developments and will know what sells well without complaints and returns. If the shop assistant seems ill-informed or off-hand on the phone, don't shop there – find someone else who is more helpful, even if it means travelling a bit further. Then grab your running mate and go shopping together.

Choose for comfort. Don't go with fixed ideas, and don't be seduced by well-known brand names into buying a shoe that is uncomfortable. What someone else is wearing may not be right for you. A while back, there was a shoe that became very popular as a 'cult' shoe because people liked the look of it – but it was a lightweight racer that was totally unsuitable for the heavier beginner.

Invest wisely. Be prepared to spend £20–£25 on your first pair of shoes, if not more. Try on all the shoes you can afford, and a few you can't. If your feet can tell the difference between a £20 and a £30 shoe it's worth shelling out a bit more – if not, you've got a bargain. At the other end of the scale, the most expensive shoes are not necessarily the best for you – comfort and fit are much more important.

Test drive. Go shopping in the socks you will wear for running (or buy your first pair in the shop) and try them on with the shoes. Try on as many different models as you can and take advantage if the shop allows you a 'test drive' in the street. After all, you are going to run on pavement and hard ground in the shoes, not stand around on fitted carpets (except perhaps in the pub afterwards!).

Size and fit. The size of your ordinary shoes is only a rough guide to the size of running shoe you will need. You may need a shoe that is a half or even a whole size larger than your normal shoes; and many shoes made outside the UK don't size up exactly with UK fittings. The shoe should fit your foot at its widest. It's a good idea to buy in the afternoon when your feet have warmed up and expanded. Try a variety of sizes and widths (women's and standard fittings). As a general guide, allow about ½in between your big toe and the end of the shoe; and do not buy a shoe if your foot overhangs the base of the shoe and bulges into the uppers.

You may well feel like Minnie Mouse in these great clodhoppers, and your sense of vanity may try and force you into smaller sizes so that your feet look smaller. Don't be tempted. These shoes are the best thing your feet could ask for (many people now wear running shoes all the time!).

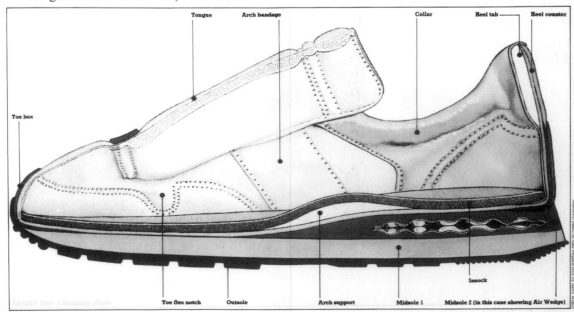

Inside the running shoe

While there should be plenty of room for your toes to move, your heels should fit snugly in the back of the shoe with no sideways movement.

Don't imagine that, like leather shoes, your running shoes can be 'broken in'. *If they don't fit in the shop, they'll never fit.*

Tread. Choose the right sole for the type of area you'll be running in. If you live in an area where most of your running is going to be on pavement or road, you may prefer a flat, wavy tread which doesn't slip on pavements and is soft and springy. If, on the other hand, most of your running is likely to be on parkland or soft ground, then you'll want a studded or waffle-soled shoe which grips on rough ground and absorbs the shock of landing on uneven ground.

Inside the shoes. Feel around inside the shoes and make sure there are no rough seams or edges which could give you blisters. You'll find an insock which smooths away most of the gaps between your foot and the shoe, and though some runners manage without socks, most of us need to avoid the friction that builds up and causes blisters. There are a number of special running socks on the market, but as long as they do not have any awkward seams across the toenails then any sport socks will do.

Shoes specially for women. Until quite recently, the only concession made to women runners was cheap trainers made in pink – shoes that were good for pushing the trolley round Sainsbury's, but not much else. Now the manufacturers are taking women runners seriously, and the choice of running shoes for women has expanded rapidly.

What's the difference? Women's feet, on average, are narrower at the heel and instep than men's, so their shoes need to be constructed slightly differently. A standard shoe may fit a woman in the toe area but not be supportive enough at the heel. Try on all the fittings available to you – men's and women's. Some women's shoes still come in feminine colours and there's no doubt that they look nice – but there's nothing feminine about muddy puddles!

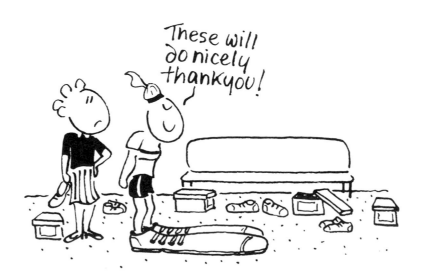

CHAPTER SIX
Your first run

On your marks . . .

While there are certainly more momentous events in a woman's life,
like losing her virginity or having a baby, your first run is
nonetheless a special occasion, and not to be rushed.

First of all, although you have the shoes, you do not necessarily need any special
clothing. Rummage around in the back of your wardrobe for any loose-fitting clothing –
slacks, T-shirt, jumper, even a dress. And if, like Belinda Charlton in Chapter Two, you
feel you need an accessory that doesn't give your new hobby away – well, yes, by all
means carry a handbag! The smart clothes come later as a reward for all your hard work.
The only other item of equipment that you or your running mate needs is a watch.

. . . get set . . .

The first thing you must do before you go out is to warm up and stretch. The warm-up
should raise your pulse a little without leaving you out of breath. You can:
* ★ switch on the radio and dance to a pop tune; or
* ★ run up and down stairs 10 times; or
* ★ skip 200 times
Try to shake the cobwebs out of your arms and legs.

PROJECT 7
THE STRETCHES

Next you must stretch your legs. It may be some time since you did any
exercise at all. When you went 'walkabout' in Chapter Five, the muscles in
your legs probably felt tight, and your joints stiff. Before *every* run, but
especially before your first run, you must pay special attention to areas of
tightness and stiffness. Getting into good habits at this stage can mean fewer
injuries later.

Let's look at the most important muscle groups in your legs, and learn to
stretch them and prepare them for running. Have your Book and pen
handy, and after each of these exercises, write down how you feel. For
example:

* ★ is that muscle very tight?
* ★ does one leg feel better or worse than the other?
* ★ did you feel better or worse after stretching?

All these stretches should be done *very slowly*, with *no* jerky movements. Don't worry if you don't stretch very far the first time.

Calf and Achilles stretch. Balance with the toes of both feet on the edge of a step. Hold on to a banister or wall if balancing is difficult. Very slowly, lean forward over your toes and let your heels drop downwards. Count to 10, then relax. Do twice more. Write down how that feels. See (a) below.

Quadriceps. Your 'quads' are the muscles at the front of your thighs. The best way to stretch them is like this. Hold on to a wall or to your running mate for balance. Standing on your right leg, bring your left leg up behind you and hold your left foot with your left hand. Count to 10, relax, and then repeat on the other foot. Do twice more on each foot. Write down how you feel. Eventually your heel should reach your bottom, but don't worry it it doesn't get there first time! See (b) below.

Hamstrings. These are the muscles at the back of your thighs. Stand on one leg and put the heel of your other foot on a wall or chair at about hip height. Keeping your back straight, bend forward very slowly from the hips. Don't lunge towards your toes! Don't worry about how far you get. Feel the stretch at the back of the raised thigh, and hold for a count of 10. Relax and repeat on the other leg. Do twice more on each leg. Write down how you feel. See (c) below.

Adductors. These are the muscles on the inside of the thigh. Stand with your feet as far apart as possible. Shift your hips to one side and then bend over the opposite leg. Count to 10, relax, and repeat on the other side. Do twice more on each side. Write down how you feel.

Don't worry if you feel terrible. You won't become flexible overnight. Some very good runners aren't flexible at all, but they still take care of their leg muscles and stretch as far as they can before every run.

. . . GO!

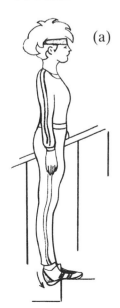 (a) 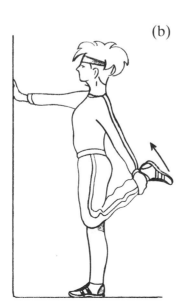 (b) 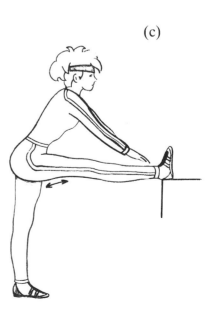 (c)

PROJECT 8

At last, you're ready to step out of the front door and run. Don't forget the front door key!

Don't set off at a hell-for-leather sprint, but as gentle a pace as you can. You and your running mate should be able to carry on a conversation. There's plenty to talk about.

I want you to run, walk and run, or just walk briskly for five minutes in any direction. As you go, think about what your body is doing, especially the feet. Go through this checklist:

★ your feet should hit the ground heel first and follow through so that you lift off on your toes

★ they should be facing forward, not inward or outward

★ let your arms hang loosely by your sides, with your hands loosely curled. No tight fists!

★ breathe normally through your mouth. In fact, try not to think about your breathing – it'll happen!

★ let the muscles of your face relax. Don't grimace

★ is there any unnecessary sideways movement? Try to iron it out. Don't let your head, arms or hips swing you from side to side

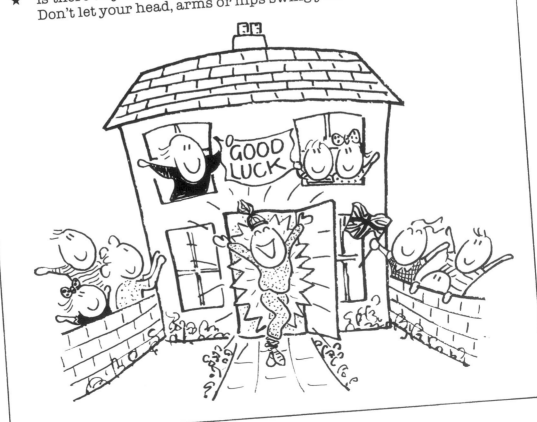

If at any time during your first run you feel giddy, lightheaded or you have pain in your chest, STOP, turn round and walk home. Sit down and wait for your pulse to go down before bathing or showering (not too hot) and relaxing. Try to explain how you feel in your Book. How long does the tightness/giddiness last?

Do the first run again after two or three days – warming up and stretching as before. Try to run or walk/run for five minutes before turning round. If the same thing happens, you should come home as before and make an appointment to see your doctor.

It is much more likely that you and your running mate will reach your five-minute goal. Remember how far you get by selecting a landmark like a lamp post, pillar box or bus stop then turn round and run, run/walk or walk back. Don't dash for home – the last part of your run should be slow and gentle.

When you get in, stretch again. It's not necessary to go through the whole sequence, but try to iron out any stiffness in particular muscles.

Then simply shake your arms, legs and head and it's time to relax. You should get out of your running clothes as soon as you can, and bath or shower. You can save time and water if you and your running mate are particularly good pals!

Dry yourself off, change into fresh clothes, splash on some cologne and sit down, Book and pen at the ready. Write down everything you can remember about your first run. If you still need some encouragement go back over Chapter One and remind yourself how other women felt on their first run. If that doesn't cheer you up, just tell yourself – it can only get better!

CHAPTER SEVEN
The rhythms of life

Up to now, I've painted a very rosy picture of running, to encourage you to think positively about your body and your fitness. And you'd be forgiven for thinking that once you become a regular runner you will float around in a constant 'high' – sun shining, birds singing, all that stuff.

It's time to bring you down to earth. The sun doesn't shine every day – and neither will you. There will be some days when you will feel simply awful. This can range from actually being ill and having to stay in bed, to a simple tired, negative feeling about your body.

I want you to start monitoring how you feel each day, listening out for changes – so that you can make the most of the times when you feel good and even use the bad times to good advantage.

Your life runs in cycles of activity, replenishment and rest, whether they are daily, weekly, monthly or yearly cycles. If you keep in touch with these cycles, you can begin to plan when you will be at your best, and run better – and you will know when to ease up and relax. Like a ploughed field, your life is full of ridges and furrows. Cutting across the ridges and furrows is hard work – running along on the top of the ridges can be fun. The simple rule is this: *Run when you're up, and rest when you're down.*

Day by day
You wake up, work, relax and sleep, During the day you eat and go to the loo a number of times. When you wake, sleep and eat will depend on your job, your family, how many hours of sleep you need, and whether you are a 'lark' or an 'owl'. 'Larks' are bright and breezy in the morning, but come 10 o'clock at night their carriages turn into pumpkins, their footmen into white mice, and they can hardly keep their eyes open. This makes them very bad company for the 'owls', who can go dancing on into the night, or sit up comforting the baby in front of the video – but hate mornings. Others, like me, can burn the candle at neither end. We all need different measures of sleep. If, for any reason, we miss out on sleep – illness in the family, changing from night to day shift, travelling across time zones or watching the Olympics from the other side of the world – we function badly the next day. Eventually we all need to catch up.

Week by week
Whenever you take the time off, the weekend should be a period for relaxation and gentle activity to shake off the cares of the week – but for how many women is that true? How many of you work *harder* on Saturdays and Sundays? Or how many of you work so hard in the week that, come the weekend, you are, as the Americans put it, 'too pooped to pop' – you haven't the energy to enjoy yourself.

Month by month
The menstrual cycle is another cycle of activity, replenishment and recovery. Every

month, you ovulate – your ovaries release a mature egg (ovum) and your womb prepares a rich lining ready for the fertilised egg – should you conceive. If you do not conceive, the lining is shed in the form of the menstrual period – in other words, your body has prepared a banquet for a VIP who hasn't turned up and the food has to be thrown away.

Periods are, without a doubt, painful, inconvenient and uncomfortable. But in many ways, we women are lucky to have them, because they tell us so much about ourselves. They tell us that we're grown-up, mature adults; that we're fertile, healthy and working normally.

The absence of periods tells us that we have not grown up yet; that we are beyond our reproductive years; that we are pregnant; or that there is something wrong that we should look into. Men do not have this handy, built-in monitoring system and as a result often push themselves too hard at times when they should be relaxing.

The contraceptive pill alters your hormonal balance so that you do not ovulate. While it leaves you secure in the knowledge that you cannot become pregnant; and your periods are lighter and more predictable, the pill masks the natural cycle, and we are still not fully aware of the long-term effects of taking it.

Some women runners take the pill continuously to postpone the menstrual period till after an important competition. This is a bit like trying to stay awake all night – eventually your body will need to catch up and when you stop taking the pill you may find the bleeding which follows is heavier and more painful. Recent research has also suggested that the pill may also make an athlete *slower* which is hardly desirable in a sport where hundredths of a second count!

Many women are changing over to other methods of contraception because they prefer the feeling of 'being in touch' with their bodies' natural cycles. At our level of running, it is better to plan your running round your menstrual cycle, not the other way about. Whichever method of contraception you use, it is important to monitor your body's changes, day by day, week by week, month by month.

Thank goodness we have left behind the Victorian era which believed that physical activity was taboo during menstruation. *Of course* you can run during your period – if you want to. Like the larks and owls of the daily cycle, it depends which type of woman you are, and the form which your monthly period takes.

Some women find that running lifts pre-menstrual tension and helps the cramps once the period has started – others feel just too awful and take two or three days' rest from running at this time of the month. Nicky Scott, of Carlisle, says 'a shorter, more gentle run through beautiful countryside calms me, and this relaxation and control alleviates period cramps. After a long hard run I have an unpleasant, light-headed, drained-out feeling.'

I belong to the other type – there are two days every month when I don't want to do *anything*, let alone run. But the exciting thing for me, and for many other women, is that running is so much better just after the period. After the activity, the replenishment and the rest, I feel a new woman altogether.

Year by year

It always beats me why people make New Year resolutions in January. Half way through the winter, when you're feeling slightly podgy from Christmas – 1 January can hardly be the best time to start changes in your life. And there is the awful burden of keeping your resolution till next 31 December. No wonder so many resolutions are broken, and so many diaries redundant by 4 January!

There are plenty of other good milestones to start from, for example:

★   the day you come back from holiday
★   your birthday
★   the first day of spring/summer/autumn/winter
★   the first day of your period
★   your child's first day back at school
★   your first day in a new job
★   the day after your last post-natal check-up
★   the day you stop breast-feeding

And you don't have to set resolutions for a whole year. Instead, try to set yourself weekly or monthly targets which you're more likely to achieve.

Keeping a diary

Your Book, in which you recorded many of your early impressions, fears and doubts about running, now becomes the most vital part of your running equipment. I want you to keep a daily record of your life – a record of which running is only a small part.

Daily record:

Every day, I want you to write the following things about yourself:

In the morning, write:
★   hours of sleep the previous night
★   resting pulse in the morning
★   the day of your menstrual cycle

In the evening, summarise:
★   how many minutes you ran for
★   where you ran
★   whom you ran with
★   the time of day you ran
★   the weather
★   what you ate
★   other sports and activities, and how many minutes you did these for
★   good feelings about the day
★   bad feelings about the day
★   your running target for tomorrow

DAILY

Sunday 9 November
hours' sleep   8
resting pulse   70
day   27 of menstrual cycle.
Ran: 60 mins, in am, with Sarah and Jo, on the common.
Felt: a bit ratty. Scraped car in car park. Cross!

Jack's birthday – celebrated with Sunday lunch at Good Companions. Too much red wine. Slept all afternoon.

Working in a plain exercise book, you don't have to worry about the length of the entries – they can be as long or as short, as detailed or as simple as you like. Some of you will want to rule your pages neatly, others of you will prefer just to let your thoughts run freely without having to pigeonhole them into a small space.

Under what you eat, I don't expect you to calorie-count every last morsel (this *isn't* a diet book!) but just give a general idea of your eating that day. For example, you may eat a big meal out one day and opt for bread and cheese the next, and this might make a difference to your running. If there's anything you're particularly trying to cut down on, like booze, chocolate or cigarettes, record your consumption of these things.

There's no need to record all the details of your menstrual cycle (unless you are using natural methods of birth control, in which case the notion of monitoring and keeping a diary won't be unfamiliar to you) but it is worth recording those times when you feel low – either in the middle of the month, when you ovulate, or in the days before and during your period.

Keep your diary on the days you don't run, too.

Say why:
★ was it a rest day?
★ were you ill?
★ or didn't you have time?

Weekly record:
At the end of each week, summarise the week's progress.

Write down:
★ total hours' sleep
★ lowest and highest resting pulse
★ the total time you ran for
★ which was your best day?
★ which was your worst day?
★ good feelings about the week
★ bad feelings about the week
★ did you feel:
  better than last week (+)?
  worse than last week (−)?
  about the same (=)?
★ target for next week

Be honest with yourself!

Weekly

Week ending Saturday 15 November
Total hours' sleep: 60½.
lowest pulse: 68

Total hours run: 2 hrs 30 min.

Good things: When I get out with the others. I feel strong and full of energy, and relaxed after. Better than last month when I wondered if I could keep up!

Bad things: Difficult to drag myself out. Too many late evenings at office. Period not *too* bad this time. Too many other things to think about. Felt very rough on Thursday.

Best day: Monday
Worst day: Thursday.

Better than last week?
No, about the same

Monthly record:
Do the same at the end of the month, going back over your daily and weekly summaries and monitoring your progress. In addition, do Project 4 – the skipping test – again and compare it with the last time you did it.

Write down:
★   total hours slept
★   highest and lowest pulse
★   best week
★   worst week
★   good feelings about the month
★   bad feelings about the month
★   the results of the skipping test alongside last month's results
★   the results (time and distance) of any fun runs or races you attempted, and how you felt about the event
★   have you noticed any regular patterns to the way you feel?
★   your weight (morning, without clothes)
★   (most important) are you still enjoying running?
★   target for next month

Monthly
Month ending 30 November

Total hours' sleep: 236
Lowest resting pulse: 67
Total hours run: 8½

Good things: I feel strong, *know* I'm getting better.
Bad things: NO WILLPOWER! Keep making feeble excuses not to run.
Best week: 16th–22nd.
Weight: 9½ stone

Skipping test:

	Last month	This month
before	72	70
after	150	148
2	130	125
5	112	110
10	72	74

progress (+)

Yearly record:

At the end of the year, your diary will run to many pages, and probably many books of daily, weekly and monthly summaries, and you'll need a bit of time to go through them all. Do the skipping test, then sit down and summarise your year.

Write down:
★ the results of your skipping test, alongside the results of the first one you did
★ total hours run
★ details of all the races and fun runs you did, and times
★ how do you feel about your progress?
   If you can honestly say you're fitter – go out and celebrate!

Yearly

Year ending 17 April 17 1985

Resting pulse last year   76   This year   61
Skipping test

before	Last year	This year
after	80	
2	160	65
5	150	140
10	140	105
	95	90
		65

Best race: Fleet ½-marathon, 1:41. Very pleased

Good things: periods lighter, feel stronger and more confident. Lost 1½ stone, kept it off.

Bad things: Granny's death knocked me sideways. Took a long time to get back.

Progress: incredible!

Your pulse tells all

Remember in Chapter Four I said that your pulse could be an important indicator of your health? As you become fitter, your resting pulse goes down, and you become more relaxed and less jittery. Keeping a daily record of your resting pulse will tell you how fit you are becoming and can sometimes help you predict the first stages of illness.

Sometimes, when you feel a little bit run down a run can brush away the cobwebs and brighten you up. Barbara Lowe, 36, from Winchester, says, 'Some days I go out feeling mentally and physically tired, and not in the mood for running at all – but by some miracle I come back refreshed and with a sense of achievement.'

That's terrific, if your weariness is more mental than physical. But supposing the tiredness is the first sign of something more serious – the early stages of flu, perhaps, or a cold, before the shivers, aches or sniffles develop. Should you run? The answer then is no, because you'll only make the cold or flu worse and possibly lay yourself open to lung infections. If you are 'going down' with something, the sooner you admit it, and rest, the sooner you will be better. Trying to 'run through' colds, coughs and flu isn't heroic. It's daft. I ran the New York Marathon in 1982 with the first signs of a cold. At the end of the race I was shivery and my body temperature had dropped dramatically; for two months afterwards I felt under the weather; and when I did run, my chest hurt. I've made the mistake – you don't have to.

But how do you know the difference between mental tiredness and the first stages of a cold? Your pulse *may* be able to help you. If, when you wake, your pulse is 10 beats or more higher per minute than the previous day, you shouldn't take any exercise that day – and you should lay off exercise till your resting pulse has gone down again. Note, though, that your pulse may well be higher in the second half of your menstrual cycle – be sure to record that in your Book.

The other sign of increasing fitness is your recovery rate. As you become fitter, and your heart and lungs get used to exercise, you recover more quickly after exercise. It's important to repeat the skipping test every month and monitor how your recovery rate is going down as you become fitter.

If you are ill, keeping a diary can be a very useful way of monitoring your illness. One of the first things a doctor will ask you, about any illness, is 'When did it start?' If you are armed with the facts and figures, you are in a much better position to help the doctor with a diagnosis and a cure. This is even more helpful if you have a complaint which recurs, because you and your doctor can work out a pattern for the problem and try and isolate any things you have done or food you have eaten which may have brought on the complaint.

Healthy eating

This isn't a diet book. I believe that regular exercise is the best way to keep your weight in check and your body in trim. But many women who have discovered the benefits of exercise have, in the process of discovering more about their bodies, become more aware of the need for a healthy, balanced diet.

Time was when 'slimming' meant cutting out bread, potatoes, rice and pasta. Reducing diets often failed because, without these, slimmers felt weak and tired, and soon started backsliding. The diet of today – which reduces the intake of fats, sugars, and salt and increases the intake of dietary fibre, is no passing fad. It ensures that active people receive all the energy they need while reducing the risk of high blood pressure, heart disease and cancer of the bowel. In other words, you should think about changing your diet for life, not till next Tuesday fortnight.

I want you to eat what you like, when you like. Have fun! But start giving some thought to healthy eating. Make changes gradually, not drastically. Set yourself monthly targets and say that, for example, you'll eat less red meat one month, more beans the next, less chocolate the next and so on. Don't forget to write down the targets and changes in your Book.

Consume more:
★   fresh vegetables

- ★ fresh fruit and unsweetened dried fruit
- ★ wholegrain cereal, pasta, rice and bread
- ★ nuts (unsalted)
- ★ beans, peas and lentils
- ★ chicken and turkey
- ★ fish
- ★ liver
- ★ yoghurt
- ★ skimmed milk
- ★ natural fruit juice
- ★ water

Consume less:
- ★ dairy produce (butter, cream, milk, cheese, eggs)
- ★ red meat (lamb, beef, pork)
- ★ cakes and biscuits
- ★ sausages and pâté
- ★ pastry and batter
- ★ rich sauces and gravy
- ★ mayonnaise
- ★ sugar
- ★ sweets and chocolate
- ★ alcohol
- ★ salt
- ★ crisps and snack foods
- ★ processed and refined food
- ★ coffee and tea

Grill, stir-fry or steam your food if possible, and avoid fried or roast foods. Treat yourself to some new cookbooks which specialise in vegetarian, fish, low-fat, low-salt or high-fibre cookery, and experiment with new dishes. Remember that any made-up canned or frozen dish may contain fat, sugar and salt, colourings and preservatives that you cannot always see or taste. If you create your own dishes from fresh ingredients, you know exactly what you're eating.

Cravings
There may be foods that you particularly feel like eating at certain times. When I get in from a long run, the first thing I feel like eating is a banana sandwich. At the back of my mind I know that bananas are a good source of potassium, which I will have lost in sweating – but that's not why I crave them. I eat them because I feel like eating them, because my body says so.

You may develop a craving for sweet things or for alcohol, just before your period. Is your period more comfortable if you indulge the cravings, or if you lay off the booze and chocolate? Experiment – then you know what to do next time. Don't feel guilty if you occasionally feel like something from the 'eat less' list!

If you drink a lot of coffee, you might not sleep very well, and you might need to drink more coffee in the morning to stay awake . . . and so on. Experiment with your coffee intake. All my routine cuppas are decaffeinated now and when I drink a really good cup of real, strong coffee I am able to enjoy it all the more, and I don't feel so muddle-headed in the mornings. But it might not work for you.

Some people are allergic to some foods – and suffer rashes, runny noses or sore eyes. You can often avoid these problems by eating unprocessed food without colouring or preservative, and keeping a record of what you eat will help you or your doctor isolate the cause of the problem.

One problem you *won't* have when you start running is constipation! The combination of exercise and a diet high in fibre will keep you astonishingly regular. Unfortunately, it's not unusual to go to the other extreme – 'rocket behind' is one Sister's polite description. Some women are afraid to run long distances because they know they will have to make embarrassing and time-wasting 'pit stops'.

This problem is probably not worth seeing your doctor about, unless you have travelled to a foreign country and/or eaten something that is contaminated. Worry only if you have acute, doubling up stomach pains, or if your stools smell unusually evil.

It is important if you have this problem to drink lots of water so that you don't become dehydrated; and to monitor your diet and your running programme to see if there are any patterns. Does it only happen at certain times of the month? Are there some foods that definitely bring it on, like cream, fruit, meat, or spicy food? Experiment with the food you eat and the time you eat it. Pat Jackson has solved her 'problem' like this: '24–48 hours before events longer than six miles, I don't eat fruit, and on the morning of the race I don't eat my usual cereal with bran – I only eat white bread toast. I seldom drink tea or caffeinated coffee.'

Biorhythms

Every daily, weekly, monthly or yearly cycle can accurately be called a 'biorhythm'. But the books you read about biorhythms concentrate on one particular theory. This is that from birth, everyone, man or woman, has three main rhythms, each with a fixed duration. Each rhythm has a positive phase, a negative phase and a critical stage when you pass from positive to negative.

★ physical cycle (23 days): in the positive phase you feel relaxed and confident about your body; in the negative phase you feel washed out and weary; and at the critical stage you are accident prone or likely to overdo exercise.
★ emotional cycle (28 days): in the positive phase you are cheerful and optimistic – it's a good time for romance and creativity; in the negative phase you are moody and critical; and at the critical stage you are touchy and over-sensitive.
★ intellectual cycle (33 days): in the positive phase you think clearly and learn fast; in the negative phase you cannot concentrate; and at the critical stage you are likely to make a hasty, wrong decision.

There is a thriving business in biorhythm watches, calculators and books. Those who believe in biorhythms have come up with all sorts of evidence to back up the theory. For example, Marilyn Monroe had just gone through a 'physical critical' and was two days away from a 'double critical' in the other two rhythms when she committed suicide. But what about all the other people born on the same day as Marilyn?

Some airlines ground pilots who are approaching biorhythmic 'criticals', though pilot error is more likely to be related to flying long hours across time zones than to the pilot's birthday.

In some ways, the theory is sound in that it says that you should monitor your good and bad days and expect to perform better at some times than others. That's exactly what I've been saying in the rest of this chapter. But I find it difficult to believe that *everyone's* physical, emotional and intellectual cycles are *exactly* the same length, and take no account of external events. As with astrology, it is very easy to find explanations which back up your beliefs. If you do believe in biorhythms or astrology, fine. But don't become hung up on them. Learn, through keeping a regular diary, to believe in *yourself*.

CHAPTER EIGHT
Building blocks

Have you ever seen two children fighting over a box of Lego? Sure as
anything, one wants to build a spaceship, the other a castle. They
start off with the same building blocks, but they have different goals,
and need different combinations of blocks to reach those goals.

I don't know you personally, but what I *do* know is that if you've got this far you now
know *yourself* much better. It is impossible to give you a personal schedule that says
that, come Hell or high water, you *must* run for 40 minutes next Thursday. Because,
come next Thursday, suppose:

★ your child is ill
★ your train is cancelled
★ you feel a bit low
★ your elderly mother is rushed off to hospital
★ there's a crisis at the office
★ an old friend, in town for only a day, calls up

Do you stick doggedly to your schedule, against all the odds, ignoring all the ups and
downs of modern life? In Chapter Seven, we looked at the body's predictable rhythms
and decided that, on the whole, it's better to swim with life's tides, not against them.
Unless you are 100 per cent organised and 200 per cent lucky, these little crises are
always going to come up.

Yet most running schedules just don't account for life's unexpected ups and downs.
They give you instructions and timetables that will never work for *you*. Like diets, they
are made to be broken. And what happens when you break a diet? You feel guilty.

That guilt can take the fun out of running. A heavy and, for you, impractical schedule
can make running just another chore to be done after you have finished the laundry.
There are two important things you must tell yourself:

★ every time you run you should enjoy yourself and achieve something – something to
   congratulate yourself on in your Book.
★ every time you don't run, you shouldn't mope and feel guilty. You probably need
   the rest, and you can put more effort into tomorrow's run.

Here, I'm simply giving you a set of building blocks, and some suggestions for putting
them together to build your own personalised schedule. Castle or spaceship, you choose,
and you build.

The foundations
On your first outing you ran, or mixed walking and running, for five minutes in one
direction and then turned round and ran or walk/ran back. Then you put your feet up

and rested for a day or two. Now it's time for your second run. When you have stretched, go out in a different direction and again keep moving for five minutes before turning for home. As before, warm down, shower, drink, and then relax and turn to your Book. Always try to keep to this after-run routine.

In your Book, record how long you went out for, and how much running you managed in the time. Did you feel better or worse than the last time?

Leave another one or two days before your third run, and then go out for five minutes in the same direction as on your first run before turning round. Did you get further than the landmark you chose on the first run? Another lamp post or tree? Or perhaps you walked less and ran more? Then you've really got something to tell your Book. You're *making progress!*

After your third run, you've finished your first week. It wasn't so hard, was it? Now is the time to plan the rest of your running life.

The basement

In your first week, did you manage to run for 10 minutes comfortably without stopping? If you're young, slim, or fit from another sport, the first week may have been quite boring for you. You already have the foundations, and you can move to the ground floor without stopping at the basement (see below). If you cannot yet run for 10 minutes without stopping, then repeat the first week until you can. You need to do this in a way that will help you to improve both the distance you run and the amount of running you do. You also need to vary your training so that it doesn't become boring for you.

Choose the three days of the second week that suit you best, making sure that you leave one or two days between each session. Say you decide to run on Sunday, Tuesday and Friday, and that you have a choice of going in two directions, north or south. Try and vary your runs like this:

SUN: north, 5mins, home, 5mins. Record how far you went (tree, lamp post, bus stop)

TUE: south, 5mins, home, 5mins. Don't concentrate on distance, but on running more and walking less.

FRI: north, 5mins, home, 5mins. Try and find a new landmark further on before turning round and coming back. Tell your Book!

The spice of life

This variation is vital if you are going to improve. Top athletes vary their training sessions like this, so that one day they run a long way slowly, the next a short distance at a faster pace. If you introduce this variety into your running, it won't be long before you find that you can run all the way for 10 minutes, without stopping to walk, and then you can proceed to the ground floor.

The ground floor

Now you're ready to start your first 20-week build-up. This is designed to build up your running, slowly but surely, in the way that best fits in with your routine. The target is that within five months of your first 'all-running' week you will be able to run a whole hour without stopping; and that, altogether, you'll be running for three hours every week, at the times that suit you best.

Some people start off by running too much, too soon, and trying to build up too quickly. All too often, that's why they become injured, or find that they are catching more colds than ever before. You have to give your body time to adjust to the new things you're asking it to do. You have to get your legs used to hitting the pavement 800 times every mile; and you have to get your heart and lungs used to working more efficiently. Think of your body as a trade union; ask it to do too much, too soon and for too little reward, and it will go on strike.

Now look at the panel.

The first 20 weeks.

Week no	Total mins	Longest run (mins)
1.	30	10
2.	33	11
3.	36	12
4.	40	14
5.	45	15
6.	50	17
7.	55	19
8.	60	20
9.	65	22
10.	70	24
11.	80	27
12.	85	29
13.	95	32
14.	105	35
15.	115	38
16.	125	42
17.	140	47
18.	150	50
19.	170	57
20.	180 (three hours)	60 (one hour)

In your first all-running week (Week 1) you ran for 10 minutes, three times in the week, a total of 30 minutes. Write up each run in your Book, and record the total minutes run in your weekly summary. Did you reach the target of 30 minutes' running? Was it all right (a + week); so-so (=) or was it a struggle (−)? If your answer is (+) or (=), go on to Week 2. If you were not happy with Week 1 go over it again till you feel you are making progress.

You'll see from the second column that in Week 2 you should run a total of 33 minutes. The figure in the third column tells you the number of minutes that your longest run of the week should be – in this case, 11 mins. You can therefore run week 2 in a number of different ways to suit your own routine:

★ 3 × 11 mins
★ 2 × 12 mins (slow) + 9 mins (fast)
★ 2 × 10 mins (steady) + 13 mins (slow)

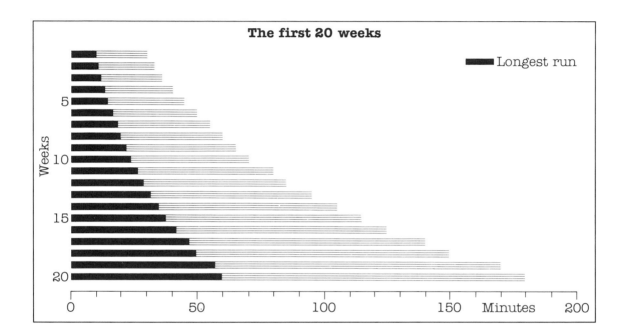

Happy? Then carry on through the schedule, moving forward a week when you record a (+) or (=) in your weekly report, and staying put when you don't feel you have made progress (−).

It's up to you to decide *when* to run, but always follow the golden rules below:

1. Run at least three times a week, every week. Any less and you are really wasting your time. When you are unfit, your body quickly forgets that you took it for a little jog a couple of weeks ago, and starts back again at square one.

2. Run no more than five times a week. Running several days in a row without rest is like trying to stay awake all night – eventually your body catches up and cries out for rest. A tired, overworked body is more likely to get injured. A rest day allows you to approach each new running day fresh and raring to go. Some people try to pack all their running into the weekend and the beginning of the week, but you are much more likely to improve if you spread the load over the whole week.

3. Never run for more than two days in a row – and never *not* run for more than two days in a row. This gives you more scope than you think! At most this means five running and two rest days a week; at least, it means three running days and four rest days. Look at the following example of three weeks for a 'maximum' runner:

SUN	MON	TUE	WED	THU	FRI	SAT
run	run	rest	run	run	rest	run
run	rest	run	run	rest	run	run
rest	run	run	rest	run	run	rest

= 14 running days

Now look at this example of three weeks for a 'minimum' runner:

SUN	MON	TUE	WED	THU	FRI	SAT
run	rest	run	rest	rest	run	rest
run	rest	rest	run	rest	run	rest
rest	run	rest	run	rest	rest	run

= 9 running days

Whichever type of runner you are, you choose the days to suit you, and space them out sensibly over the week.

From running three days a week, you can build up to four and then five days when you feel like it, as long as you complete that week's recommended total, and as long as your longest run is at least as long as recommended in the third column.

4. Vary your running. Don't go plodding out the same boring old course at the same speed every time. You'll bore yourself to death, and your improvement won't be as rapid as if you treat yourself to a varied diet. After all, however much you like, say, spaghetti Bolognese, you don't eat it every night of the week, do you? We'll look at some examples of planning your running 'menu' a bit later on.

5. If, at any time you find it's a struggle and you fall short of your target total, don't despair. There may also be weeks in which you are ill or injured, or on holiday, and you don't run at all. If this happens, it's not necessary to go right back to the beginning. For every week you don't run, or run a little but fail to reach the target total of minutes go back the same number of weeks in your schedule – for example, if you are ill for Weeks 9 and 10 you should try and go over Week 7 again, and repeat it if necessary till you feel confident and fit enough to go on to Week 8.

You will only need to go right back to the beginning if you are out of action for several months, for example if you have an accident or operation.

6. However good you feel at the end of each week, don't be tempted to jump *ahead* in the schedule. Over-enthusiasm can lead to injury.

As you begin to plan each new week in your Book, you'll see just how flexible this schedule is.

The first floor

Your first five months as a runner are the most exciting, because this is the time when you will make the most noticeable progress, even if your 20-week schedule is longer and more drawn out because of the odd problem you haven't been able to anticipate. When you have completed this schedule, you have climbed the stairs and you are now ready to explore the first floor of this spaceship or castle you are building. Let's look again at what you have achieved.

You are now running for three hours a week, and one outing is a continuous run of an hour. Five months ago you could barely run for 10 minutes at a time! So it's time to sit down and tell the Book how you feel about that. Allow several pages for backslapping and congratulation – ask your Sister or your family what they think about your achievement.

Has it been easy to fit running in with your life? Can you still honestly say that you are enjoying it? What have been the major benefits so far? How about going out for a slap-up meal and cracking open a bottle of something festive?

Then I want you to have a gentle week, either not running at all, or running just a little, and decide what you want to do next. Do you want to:

★ give up here and now? Really, if you've reached this far, I don't see that happening.
★ maintain your current level of running? It may well be that three hours a week is all you have time for. Well, that's more than enough. I hope by now you've come to reap some of the benefits mentioned in earlier chapters – weight loss, more energy, better sleeping patterns, giving up smoking. Three hours a week is quite enough to keep all these good things going for you, without biting too deep into your domestic, work and leisure routine. Now you're running confidently, you can start to make the best of the running you do.
★ perhaps you're completely bitten by the bug and would like to put more time into your running so that you can think about serious racing over 10 miles, half-marathon and perhaps even the marathon – but before you try and increase the time run, I do suggest that you spend some time improving the quality of your running.

Running menus

Pounding round and round the same route, at the same speed, every time you run is not only boring, it doesn't do anything to help you improve. You may have heard other runners talking about 'repetitions', 'intervals', 'LSD' and even something that sounds rather rude called 'fartlek'. All these things, and others, are techniques that top athletes use – but they're just as valuable for you. Let me explain some of these terms.

LSD. This is short for long, slow distance – which means what it says. You run a long way at a very, very easy pace to build up endurance. You can tell if the pace is right by trying the 'talk test'. If you can't keep up a normal conversation with your running partner, you're going too fast. You should aim to do at least one long slow run a week which is about a third of the total time you spend running – so if you run for three hours a week, your longest run should be at least an hour long. As you can carry out a sensible conversation, LSD can be very sociable running. In the right company, and if you choose a scenic route, LSD can be terrific fun.

Interval training. This isn't usually so much fun, but it's good for you! The idea is that you run a short distance (200–800m) flat out; then walk or jog to recover and then run fast again. To begin with, it may take you a long time to recover, but as your heart gets used to the bursts of effort, your recovery time will become shorter. This is what you should be aiming for. Don't try to make the fast bursts faster or longer but keep them the same and aim to bring your recovery time down. Interval training is usually done timed, on a track.

Fartlek. This means 'speed-play' in Swedish. Like interval training, it helps you build up speed but it is more fun. Out on a fartlek run you'll set yourself a target that is 200–800m away (like a lamp post, bus stop or pillar box) and run at a faster pace towards it. Then you walk or jog gently till you feel it's time to tackle another target. This is even more fun if you're out running with someone else as you will encourage each other to keep going, and you can run with people of different standards. The speedy ones will work harder, but they can jog back to you, so you'll not be left behind.

Repetitions. 'Reps' are no fun at all – they're agony – but there's no doubting that they will help you build up speed. The idea is that you go out and run a fast one- or two-mile lap and time it; then rest for up to 10 minutes and do it again. And again. And a fourth and final time. Aaargh!

Hills. A lot of people complain that when they go out of their front doors 'the only way is up!' They are lucky, because they are already reaping the benefits of hill training. When they come to race on the flat they will be at an advantage.

You should try and include some hills in all your training runs, at whatever speed, though I appreciate that's difficult if you live in East Anglia! If a hill threatens you, tell yourself that you can relax when you reach the top – *not before*! When you're there and ready to go downhill, take a deep breath, drop your arms, stick your chest and chin out (like Eric Liddell in *Chariots of Fire*) and *float*.

Don't attempt any speed work (intervals, fartlek, repetitions, hills) if you don't feel 100 per cent. If you feel slightly under the weather, but not bad enough to stop you running, opt for a slow run, because if you do have a cold coming on, or a niggling injury, speed work isn't going to help it.

Always remember your pre-run stretching routine. A fast run on tight, unstretched muscles is the surest way to become injured. Warm up, stretch, jog gently, then stretch again before any of these speed sessions. At the end, stretch and jog gently to warm down.

Supplementary benefits

Many of the women you met in Chapter One keep fit in other ways, and the confidence that running has given them has encouraged them to take up other sports. But I have women writing to me to explain, almost apologetically, that they have substituted a dance class for one of their running sessions; that they cycle to and from work and so don't feel like running so much; or that while on holiday, they swam every day but didn't do any running.

Good for them! I believe it's very important not to become so single-minded about your running that you don't have time for the other activities that you enjoy.

Although running is an excellent way of keeping the heart and lungs fit, it does only exercise a limited range of muscles. And its repetitive nature means that, however cautious you are in building up your schedule, you are still open to the risk of injury.

So start to think about a balanced diet of fitness activities that take the repetitiveness out of running and develop other areas of skill.

For some of you, running may be the first sport you have ever tackled and achieved. With your new-found confidence you might feel like taking up something new – like a team or racket game. Others of you may have dabbled in sport or dance before but not kept it up for lack of energy and enthusiasm. The fitness you build up from running may vitally change your attitude to that other sport – so go back and look at it afresh.

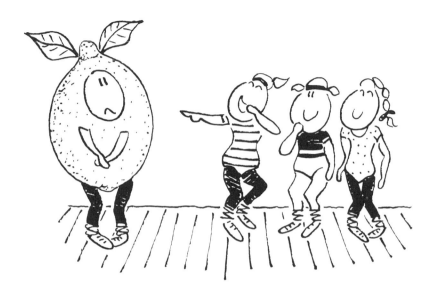

Aerobic dance

I have mixed feelings about 'aerobics'. On one hand I think it's terrific that the likes of Jane Fonda and Jackie Genova have encouraged millions of women to think positively about their bodies and about exercise. But I don't believe that it's the type of exercise that appeals to, or is suitable for, every woman.

Me, for example. Though fit, I am uncoordinated, and, without my glasses, incredibly stupid. If the teacher says 'left' my right side responds; if she says 'count to 10' I will count to 11 – if I've heard her, which isn't always possible over the blare of loud music. Though confident in shorts, I feel a real lemon in a leotard. I'm sure I'm not alone.

That said, aerobic dance may be more your bag than running. A good class will give you a balanced programme of exercise of which the aerobics is usually only a small part – the rest is taken up with developing suppleness and strength in all the muscle groups; and there should also be a relaxation session.

So aerobic dance is valuable as conditioning for the whole body. Unfortunately, there are quite a few 'cowboy' teachers around keen to make a profit from aerobics, teaching without qualifications and without taking an interest in their pupils' health or requirements. I hope this book has taught you more about your body and about its warning signs to recognise who is and who isn't a good aerobics teacher.

On your first visit to the class, a good teacher should:

★ take the time to find out a bit about you and your fitness – for example whether you smoke, take the pill, have high blood pressure or a history of heart disease and how much exercise you are already taking

★ advise you on footwear

★ ask you why you want to do her classes – if there are any particular aspects of your fitness that you'd like to develop
★ put the beginners to the front of the class and keep a special eye on them to make sure that all the exercises (especially those which put pressure on the back and abdomen) are being done properly
★ not force you through pain, but give you the option of stopping when you are either out of breath or in pain
★ not encourage you to keep up with more experienced pupils.

If she does a 'slow stretch' or yoga class it may be worth going to that instead. You will learn co-ordination and control and become flexible in slow motion without having to keep up with fast music, and you are less likely to become injured. Although the exercises are slow, they work every part of the body, and come the relaxation at the end you may well be ready to fall asleep – I usually am!

Other aerobic sports

Cycling and *swimming* are both excellent for heart and lung fitness and are a good part of an all-round fitness programme. Unlike running, they don't send shock waves through your body with every stroke or downpedal. They are essential parts of your training schedule if you cannot run for any reason. For example, women in the later months of pregnancy often switch to swimming or stationary cycling because the baby is putting too much pressure on the spine and on the bladder, and thus makes running very uncomfortable. If you are injured, treading water or 'running' in the swimming pool are good ways of recovering fitness before you go back to pounding the roads. Cycling exercises different muscles of the leg and swimming works the upper body too. *Rowing*, either on a rowing machine or, better still, the real thing, exercises heart, lungs, arms, legs and abdomen, but can damage the back if not done properly – ask a rowing coach or gym instructor to supervise your first efforts.

Nordic (cross-country) skiing

This is becoming a popular holiday sport because, unlike downhill skiing, cross-country is a form of running on skis which goes both uphill and downhill. The skis are longer than downhill skis, and you are only attached to them by the toes, so that your feet are more flexible. In a day's Nordic skiing, you can pick up good speed and take in some breathtaking scenery! *Walking* is good for scenery, too, and if you've had a hard week there's nothing to beat a quiet weekend briskly walking along one of Britain's many long distance footpaths.

Upper body work

Runners usually neglect the upper body and wonder why they have back pain, neck pain or tension in the shoulders. Swimming, rowing and weight training can help to tone up the upper body and get you thinking about ironing out those pains and tensions.

Weight training

Not that heavyweight stuff you see those big guys doing in the Olympics, and it won't give you bulging biceps or big thighs. Weight training can help you tone up and strengthen specific areas of the body. Improvement comes not by lifting heavier and heavier weights, but by increasing the number of times the individual exercises are done ('repetitions' or 'reps').

Racket sports
Squash is the most aerobic of the racket sports, but you will be a better player if you combine squash with running. *Tennis*, *badminton* and squash are all very good sports for developing eye-hand co-ordination and, though hectic, give you some time to think about your stroke and your tactics and how they can be improved.

Team sports
Perhaps your school days have put you off team sports for life. But now, as a runner, you can call yourself a sportswoman – and you might want to think again about playing *basketball*, *hockey*, *lacrosse*, *volleyball* – and relishing the importance of being part of a team.

Mind and body
I would fully recommend *yoga* (especially the very physical Iyengar yoga) to runners, men and women. You will learn to stretch, to breathe, to think about your body, and you will learn to relax. Although in yoga it doesn't often look as though you're doing very much, you can come out feeling quite puffed and invigorated because all your mental and physical energy has been directed inwards. The martial arts (for example, *judo, t'ai chi and karate*) can also teach you a lot about the relationship between mind and body.

Balance/skill/excitement
Now you've got the confidence – try *windsurfing* or *downhill skiing* or even *hang-gliding*. Live a little!

CHAPTER NINE
A day at the races

Racing. The very word may turn you right off. The idea of pitting your new-found strength against others may fill you with horror. By its very nature, it implies that someone has to be first and someone has to be last. I think I can guess which end of the race you're worried about!

The wonderful thing about running competitively is that you can often find yourself in the same races as the stars. I've run a marathon with Grete Waitz, of Norway, who was the first woman to break 2½ hours for the marathon, and I have raced at many distances with Joyce Smith, Priscilla Welch and Sarah Rowell who represented Britain in the first Olympic marathon for women in Los Angeles in 1984.

I'm no great threat to their supremacy, however, for my marathon time is nearly an hour slower. There is no other sport in which the untalented can share the same arena as the best. Can you imagine having the chance to play three sets against Martina Navratilova on the hallowed green of Wimbledon? Never in a million years.

Of course, someone has to be last. The first year the Avon 10-mile race was held that honour went to Kate Symonds, of Barnet, who finished in 1 hour 43 minutes.

It wasn't so bad for Kate after all. For one thing, she won a television set in the raffle – for another, she's never been last since. In every race she tackled after that she promised herself she would come next from last, then third from last, then fourth, and so on. The following year she ran the Avon 10 more than 15 minutes faster and was nowhere near last! 'The experience wasn't demoralising at all,' she says. 'I feel I conquered the distance.' She feels she gathered strength from the people who had to drop out from the encouragement and the cheers she received from the crowd, and from the really satisfying feeling of keeping going.

In Chapter One we met Sheila Giles, who makes coming last her hobby, and loves it – for she always raises the loudest cheers. Brenda Forbes brought up the rear of a women's 10 km (6.2 mile) race in Wolverhampton. Eight hundred yards from the finish, she was saying 'I'm so ashamed . . . I'm so ashamed.' After the finish she was as bright as a button, for she, too, won the loudest cheers of the day.

You may simply want to run for fitness and fun, but most women find that setting themselves the target of competition helps them improve; it gives them confidence as they realise they're not as slow as they thought; and it makes sure they meet lots of other women of the same standard with whom they can swap tips, share ideas, and say 'see you next time'.

However, it's important that you don't set your sights too high too soon. If you fail, you'll lose confidence. You may also fall into the trap of building up too quickly – and thus find you are injured by the time race day comes along.

Here's a guide to different types of running event, and when you can realistically expect to be able to tackle them.

Under six miles
You should start tackling fun runs, relays and handicaps as soon as you can! Even if you have to walk some of the way first time around, they'll give you some measure of your ability – and bags of confidence. The biggest event in the fun run calendar is the *Sunday Times* National Fun Run, first held in 1978. The Fun Run is 4 km or 2½ miles long, on grass and paths in London's Hyde Park. This event now attracts over 30,000 people each year. They don't all run at once, but in groups subdivided into age and sex. The day starts at 10.00am and finishes at 5.00pm after the mass jog – when everyone can run together, and many people do so in fancy dress, or with very small children. If you can travel to London it's a day out to remember – it happens in September every year, and details appear in the *Sunday Times* from about May onwards.

Many jogging clubs now organise short fun runs, handicaps or relays. They are usually arranged so that there are prizes for people of all standards – rewarding your effort and improvement rather than your actual ability. A handicap works like this. The first time around, everyone runs the same distance, starting off at the same time. Some speedy bloke wins, and leaves you trailing. However, the next time, the race is arranged so that you start off ahead of him, and he has to work very hard to catch you up. If you keep in front of the faster people all the way round, you're the winner!

This works particularly well in one of the clubs I run with, the Stragglers, based in Kingston-upon-Thames. Every month the Stragglers handicap pits fast men against beginner women. Who wins? Usually the women, because they are the ones who have made most improvement over their time for the previous month. It is a lot easier to improve a slow time by five minutes than it is a fast time by five seconds!

In relay races, you feel a responsibility to other members of the team. You can't let them down, so what do you do? You go faster! At the end of the race you can celebrate and applaud your team's effort – and your own contribution to it.

All these short events are meant to be taken lightheartedly (though some people contest the *Sunday Times* Fun Run in deadly earnest!). Often your husband and family can take part as well. One recent arrival to this country (from the USA, of course) is the Twosome, which you run with a male partner – your scores are added up, and the top twosome wins.

Six to nine miles
The most common race in this family is the 10 km – 10,000 metres or, in old money, 6.2 miles. You can expect to run 10 km after about three months' training, when you've managed a long run of between 45 and 60 minutes. Expect to run your first 10 km in around an hour, and then see how much you can improve the next time. The 10 km is without a doubt my favourite distance, and many of the Sisters agree with me.

'It's short enough to run hard all the time, long enough to make use of my stamina' (Fiona Nixon, Tonypandy); 'It's just the right distance to try a little bit faster than usual' (Maria Williams, Harlow); 'I really haven't time to train for longer distances' (Jean Trahearn, Lincoln); 'I can finish feeling good, but not exhausted' (Christine Hastings, Bromley); 'It's long enough to be fast but not so far that you drag around for hours' (Christine Harrison, Basildon); 'It's not too far, but I need two miles to get going' (Daphne Rowland, Ipswich); 'I can race all the way – anything over, I mess up the pace' (Margaret Robinson, Troon); 'Long enough for me to have a chance of doing well in my age group and short enough to be enjoyable' (Jean Kanssen, Virginia Water); 'I soon had enough experience to know that I could catch up with those who started off too fast!' (Patricia Hardy, Sutton Coldfield); 'It doesn't mean having several days' rest to get over it' (Anne Graham, Gosport).

10 miles

I'm not as keen on racing 10 miles, though it's a nice round number to aim for. I tend to set off as though I was running a 10 km and struggle the last four miles. But other women like the 10 miles because it's not as fast as the 10 km: 'It's easier to chicken out of really pushing myself to the limits, whereas in shorter distances I feel more of an obligation to hurt' (Kay Gillespie, Greenwich); 'A good satisfying distance – there are tactics as well as strength involved' (Viv Williamson, Colindale); 'My knees won't stand up to more miles in training for longer distances' (Sheila Thompson, Woodstock).

Ten miles is a more traditional distance for the hardened 'club' runner, and it's possible if you're a relative newcomer to find yourself in the wrong kind of race – one where the organisation is only geared to the faster runners, and where the marshals look disapprovingly at their watches as you jog past with a lap to go – almost as if they're dying to go home for their tea.

It is always best to ask advice from an experienced runner on choosing a 10, and this is where joining a club can be helpful. Women-only 10s, or races which exclude faster runners (for example, the Masters and Maidens races in Surrey) are geared towards veterans and women, and there are certain qualifying times that you must fall *below* in order to run. These lower-key races are recommended.

To be at your best for your first 10M, you should have been running for five months, with a longest run of 1:30.

Half-marathon

This is another popular distance for newer runners, and perhaps the shape of races to come. You can expect to run a half-marathon (13 miles, 192½ yards) after six months' training with a longest run of 1:40. I like 'halves' because, unlike in my disastrous 10-milers, I manage to pace myself sensibly from the start, and then I can pick up speed in the last 3.1 miles. Women who like the half-marathon are often concerned that they lack speed over shorter distances. 'I suffer from breathing problems if running at speed. A 10-miler is a sprint to me!' (Marion Skett, Tunbridge Wells); 'It's far enough for speed merchants to tire so that I can catch them' (Linda Reed, Warminster); 'Long enough to be a decent challenge but not impossible' (Diana Mealing, Bristol).

Marathon

There's no doubt about it, the marathon's a tremendous experience. There's little can beat, for me, the anticipation of coming round the corner to see Tower Bridge ahead of you, marking the halfway point of the London Marathon – and then what seems like half a lifetime later crossing Westminster Bridge at the finish; or in New York, coming off the rather lonely Queensboro Bridge which links the boroughs of Queens and Manhattan to find what seems like the whole world ready to greet you with balloons, claxons, and the human voice. They could skip over to Central Park a few blocks away and see the winner coming in, but no, they stay to see *you*.

Everyone who has done a marathon has their own memories, their own experiences, their own 'highs'. 'The greatest feeling of triumph, exhilaration and well-being ever felt' (Julie Roberts, Liverpool); 'There's time to be sociable and get into my stride. I also like the people, the cheers, the encouragement . . .' (Joyce Smith, Wimbledon); 'I like the gradual start and the lovely peaceful feeling that no-one else will bother me for the next 26-odd miles' (Frances Classon, Clwyd).

But 26 miles and 385 yards is a *very long way*. It is the distance from Windsor Castle to the old White City stadium in London's Shepherds Bush which, sadly, was pulled down at the end of 1984. The exact distance was decided in 1908 when the Olympic Games were held in London and Queen Alexandra insisted that the competitors finished in front of the Royal Box – hence the odd number of extra yards.

Think about it next time you're in the car. It's approximately the distance from London to Guildford; from Exeter to Lyme Regis; from Swansea to Merthyr Tydfil; Birmingham to Rugby; Stratford-upon-Avon to Cheltenham; Dundee to Montrose.

And there's no way you can short-cut your training for the marathon. If you tried to run 26 miles without any preparation, you would do your body a lot of damage, and you would place a strain on the first aid and medical services.

How different is marathon training?

In Chapter Eight, I suggested that you progress gradually up to three hours' running a week, dropping back when you didn't feel so positive about your running, and pressing on when you did.

Three hours a week is quite enough to achieve and maintain fitness, and enjoy yourself. I don't think you should think about entering a marathon until you have reached this target, and have been running regularly for about a year. You should also have tackled a few races, including the half-marathon, to adjust to the feeling of pacing yourself, and of running with lots of other people.

Then you have to ask yourself: Can I fit *another* three hours' running into my life? That may sound fairly easy, but it's not as easy as fitting in the first three. The increase in training increases the risk of injury. Instead of feeling bright as a button and raring to go, you may start feeling tired and run down. People will tell you you're looking ill, when you've never felt fitter in your life. There may have to be some sacrifices in home and social life. If you don't have the full support of your family and friends, training may be an uphill struggle. I well remember those cold midweek evenings, when, just about to go out for a 10-mile run, someone would call up and say, 'Fancy a beer, Ali?' Should I decline the invitation and risk losing a valued friend, or should I give in, and risk losing valuable training miles? The marathoner often becomes impatient when ill or injured and often starts again too soon. In short, running stops being fun.

I know. I'm being a real wet blanket and painting as miserable a picture of marathon training as I can. But if you've read this far, you're clearly determined, so it's time to start thinking positively with a few tips on marathon training.

You must still follow all the guidelines in Chapters Seven and Eight: not running every day; varying the type of running you do; not moving forward in your schedule if you fail to reach last week's target; not running when you are ill. To reach your target of six hours a week, add 15 minutes a week to the previous week's total. Ten of these should be added to your longest run of the week, so that you end up with a longest run of three hours two weeks before your chosen marathon date. Then you should wind down for two weeks before your marathon, relaxing and just running a little when you feel like it.

Marathon training schedule
(hours and minutes)

Week	Week's total	Longest run
1.	3:00	1:00
2.	3:15	1:10
3.	3:30	1:20
4.	3:45	1:30
5.	4:00	1:40
6.	4:15	1:50
7.	4:30	2:00
8.	4:45	2:10
9	5:00	2:20
10.	5:15	2:30
11.	5:30	2:40
12.	5:45	2:50
13.	6:00	3:00
14.	3:00	1:30
15.	3:00	1:00

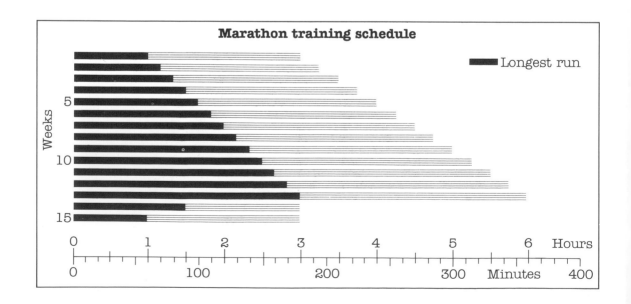

PROJECT 9
SETTING YOURSELF A TARGET

In Chapter Eight I said that you all will have different goals, and different ways of reaching those goals, according to your age, ability, and the time you are prepared to devote to your training. Now I want you to identify those goals. Your next step is to buy a copy of *Running* magazine.

Turn to the *Running Events* section. This lists road races all over Britain for the current and following month. Find a race (any distance) that you like the look of, that isn't too far away from your home. Write to the organiser, enclosing a stamped addressed envelope, and simply ask for details of time and date of the race, and where it starts and finishes. *Then go and watch it!*

Wallow in the atmosphere of the start and finish, cheer loudly for the leaders and even more loudly for the tailenders. Are there women like you in the race? Try and talk to them afterwards. Congratulate them, ask them how they feel about the race, and ask them what their next target is. It might be a race that you can do. Don't be afraid to ask their advice. Write down your impressions in your Book.

Then find a race or fun run in your area which you think you are ready to *run*. Write to the organiser, enclosing a stamped, self addressed envelope, and ask:

★   is the race suitable for your standard?
★   what is the *slowest* time acceptable?
★   are there adequate changing and toilet facilities for women?
★   do you have to be a member of a club?

If you get no answer, or a snotty answer, it may not be your sort of race. Look for another one. When you have decided on your target, write it down in your Book and work out how much running you are going to do in the weeks between now and the event. Remember that for a 10km your longest run should be 45—60 minutes; 10 miles 1—1:30 and half-marathon 1:30—1:40.

If you eventually want to run a marathon, look in *Running* at the events listed for *this* year. As before, choose one in your area and go along to watch it and talk to the runners afterwards. If you like what you see, promise yourself, 'That's the one I'll do next year,' and start gently increasing your training straight away.

Branching out

Ultra distance. For some women, even 26.2 miles is not enough! Christine Barrett, 36, an aerobics teacher from Brockworth, is one of those who prefers to go on for 30, 40, 50,

100 miles; to race for 24, 48 hours or even (no kidding) six days. This is called 'ultra distance running' and is one area in which women can shine, because ultra runners are the sort of people who lack basic speed but have the stamina and the determination to plod on and on . . . and on.

Going further

For some women, even 26.2 miles is not enough! Christine Barrett, 36, an aerobics teacher from Brockworth, is one of those who prefers to go on for 30, 40, 50, 100 miles; to race for 24, 48 hours or even (no kidding) six days. This is called 'ultra distance running' and is one area in which women can shine, because ultra runners are the sort of people who lack basic speed but have the stamina and the determination to plod on and on . . . and on.

'Six-day' racing became a popular sport in Victorian times and has recently been revived. In this, the competitors run or walk round and round a track between noon on Sunday and noon the following Saturday – stopping when they want to eat, sleep, go to the loo, have their legs massaged or their blisters lanced. Sounds crazy, but Christine Barrett loves it. She set a new women's world record for the distance in 1984 (it's since been broken again by Eleanor Adams) of 421 miles (approximately the equivalent of running from Gloucester to Middlesborough and back) and holds many other ultra distance world records.

Triathlon

Christine Barrett is also a fan of the triathlon, a new sport which combines running with cycling and swimming, though not in that order – the swimming comes first, the running last. She has taken part in one of the hardest endurance events in the world, the Iron Man Triathlon in Hawaii, where you swim for 2.4 miles, cycle 112 miles and *then* run a 26.2 mile marathon!

Christine had not been a sportswoman all her life, though she has danced and taught ballet. She gave up smoking and took up jogging in 1979 to regain some fitness after a skiing accident. Then she cracked her skull in a bike accident, but carried on her training as soon as she was recovered, running her first marathon in 1981.

She trains when she feels like it, rests when she doesn't, teaches aerobics five times a week and doesn't suffer too many running injuries. The kinds of events she tackles are hard, mentally and physically, but she is always photographed with a smile on her face. Her refreshing attitude to endurance events is that 'when they stop being fun, I'll stop doing them'.

The Iron Man Triathlon is no event for the ordinary jogger looking for a bit of adventure. It requires talent and dedication (you can catch up on ability later, as Christine found). However, the 'short' triathlon is fast gaining popularity. Swimming 800m–one mile, cycling 25–40 miles, running 5–13 miles is within more people's grasp.

The triathlon season is short in Britain because most of the swims take place in open water, and there are only a few months of the year when the lakes and rivers are warm enough! Training for a short triathlon is a good all-round fitness programme, and is probably the reason why Christine has the stamina to run a six-day race without all the injuries that go with a running-only programme.

Christine Barrett smiling after 23 hours on the track
at Costello Stadium, Hull, July 1984 (Richard Kemp)

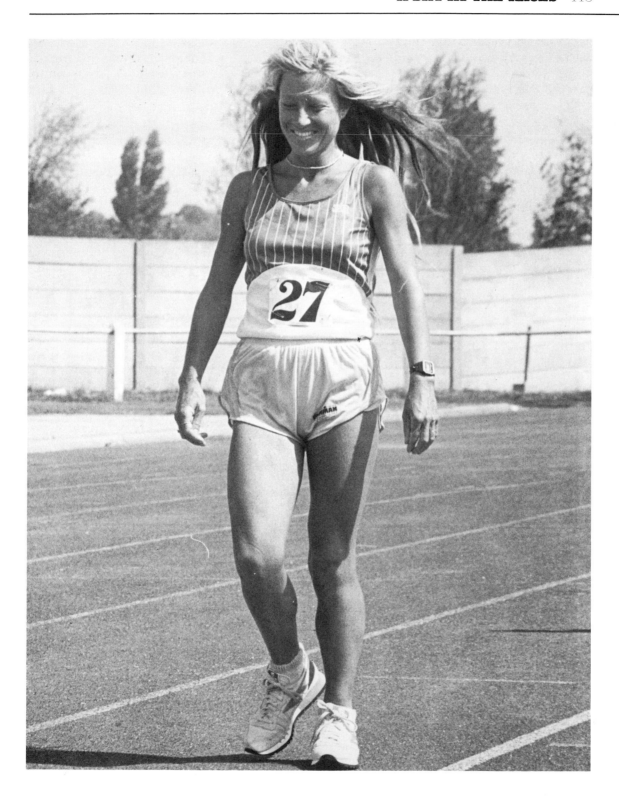

Off the beaten track

Up to now, I've concentrated on road running. That's where the running 'boom' has really made its mark. But Britain has acres of open spaces – forest, moorland, parkland, fells and commons – to explore. You won't, it's true, run so fast on rugged country, but you can build up stamina, get away from the traffic and enjoy the scenery.

Orienteering is often called 'the thought sport'. It is a popular sport with families because events are graded for age groups from under 10 to over 60 – boys and girls, men and women. Armed with map, compass and punch card, and with your legs covered because occasionally it can be a bit brambly, the aim is to navigate yourself as quickly as you can between a series of control points, where your card is punched to confirm that you've been there.

Orienteering is an excellent way of seeing the countryside and learning to combine the mental skill of map-reading with your running ability. No two events are ever the same – you may trail in hopelessly last one week, when both your concentration and your speed have let you down. The next, you get all your bearings right *and* your running feels good – and you are well placed in your age group. The mental concentration often means that you forget how far you are running. Courses are from 2 to 12 km long, but you often run much further!

Hashing. I'm hopeless with maps. Much as I love rough-terrain running, I'm unable to orienteer my way out of a paper bag. However, I do have a loud voice and a partiality for best bitter, essential qualifications for 'hashing'. Nothing to do with either marijuana or corned beef, this variation of running started in the 1930s in Malaysia, among a group of expatriate Englishmen who organised a paper chase after rather a boozy party. Until quite recently it's been rather a masculine pastime, but now women are welcome at most hashes, and it's a very good social running because the fast men aren't always the first home.

Hashing is basically foxhunting with the benefit of neither fox, horse, nor hounds. Experienced (and environmentally responsible) trail layers lay a trail of flour or sawdust over a 4–8 mile course, taking in as many ups, downs, puddles and brambles as they can find. They also lay false trails! The pack follows, and the faster runners go on ahead to the first checkpoint. As the slower runners catch up, the others go looking in all directions for the trail to begin again, and when they have done so, they shout, 'On, on,' and go off again, with the pack in pursuit. They may find they have chosen the false trail, in which case the language is usually unrepeatable. There's a lot of shouting involved – to make sure that those in front are still following the trail, and that those behind are still following you. Fast runners who have gone off on false trails end up sprinting to catch up, while slower runners can take a breather at each checkpoint. Afterwards, the hash usually retires to a real ale pub.

Cross-country. Until recently cross-country was only really open to a hardened few who had been running for athletics clubs all their lives. But why should they have all the fun of getting muddy? Now there are a number of open events every winter which welcome runners of all standards to run over marked courses from 3 to 5 miles long. You'll feel very proud of yourself as you tuck into a Thermos of tea afterwards, for while cross-country is hard work, it is also exhilarating, and a good way of shaking off the blues of a winter afternoon. You'll need a pair of shoes with more grip than your road shoes, and you mustn't worry about getting them – or the rest of you – dirty once a week. If your husband and kids can come home on Saturday with dirty kit, so can you!

Fell running. Fell running has its roots in the Lake District, but is now practised widely in the North of England, in Scotland and parts of Wales. A good fell runner doesn't just race to the top of the fells quickly – descending quickly and fearlessly is the important skill. Very few women run the fells, which is a pity, but if you live in the right place and have reached the right level of running, it's worth a try. The Fell Runners Association (address on page 124) publishes an annual calendar of events helpfully classified by distance, terrain, ability and conditions. You have to be very hardy and very experienced to tackle a race marked 'navigational skills in mist required'.

On the track

In Chapter Eight we looked at the value of running timed intervals on the track for building up speed. Track running is not everyone's cup of tea – most of us suffer it for, like evil-tasting medicine, we feel it is doing us good! But suppose you're one of those people who enjoys 400m, 800m, 1,500m or 3,000m and for whom track work is not just a means to an end? Then you should start looking out for 'open graded' meetings – track events held throughout the summer at which you can run against others of a similar standard at the shorter track distances. If you want to pursue a track career, though, it is best to join an athletics club which has the coaching facilities to set you on your way.

CHAPTER TEN
Clubbing together

You are now running between two and three hours per week. You may have run your first race; if not, it is not long off the horizon. What next? Do you and your running mate just keep plodding on together for mile after mile? If the answer is yes, that's fine. You are lucky if you are evenly paced and have similar commitments and ambitions – running together is still the right thing for you. But it's time for both of you to think about widening your horizons and joining a club – or starting one up if there's nothing suitable in your area.

'Runners are such friendly and trusting people,' says Lynne Butler of Woodford Green. Lynne joined Essex Ladies and 'it was the best thing I have ever done. Imagine how proud my parents are that their gawky asthmatic daughter trains alongside members of the British team!'

Like Lynne, joining a club may be the best move you make. In the company of different runners, you will improve by leaps and bounds; you'll widen your circle of friends; you'll find out about races (some clubs organise travel to faraway places to run races – and have a good time in the process); and you'll pick up all sorts of useful hints about shoes and equipment.

But there are pitfalls. The nearest club for you might not meet at a convenient time – and it may not have other people like you in it. There's nothing more demoralising than going along to a club for the first time and finding that you're the only woman/beginner/ over 40 (or, heaven help you, all three) there. So it pays to do a little bit of research before you turn up, like I did, and find everyone disappearing over the horizon before you've even been introduced.

There are three different types of club.

Athletics clubs or harriers. These are the traditional clubs, which nurture top athletes like Kathy Cook, Tessa Sanderson, Wendy Sly and Shirley Strong. They regularly field teams for track and field competition in the summer and cross-country in the winter.

'Traditional' can sometimes mean 'old-fashioned'. Some clubs haven't woken up to the fact that more and more men and women, of different ages and abilities, want to run. They only want talented, committed athletes. In a club like this you may find yourself totally out of your depth and think you're in another sport altogether – or you may feel at home from your first visit. Most athletics clubs are affiliated to the Amateur Athletic Association and the Women's AAA or their regional organisations.

A Day at the Races
– before the start –

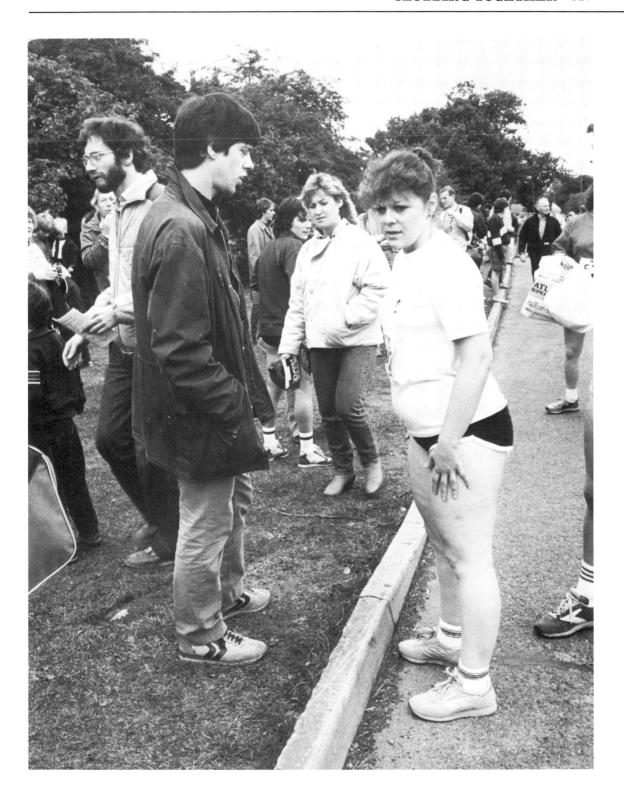

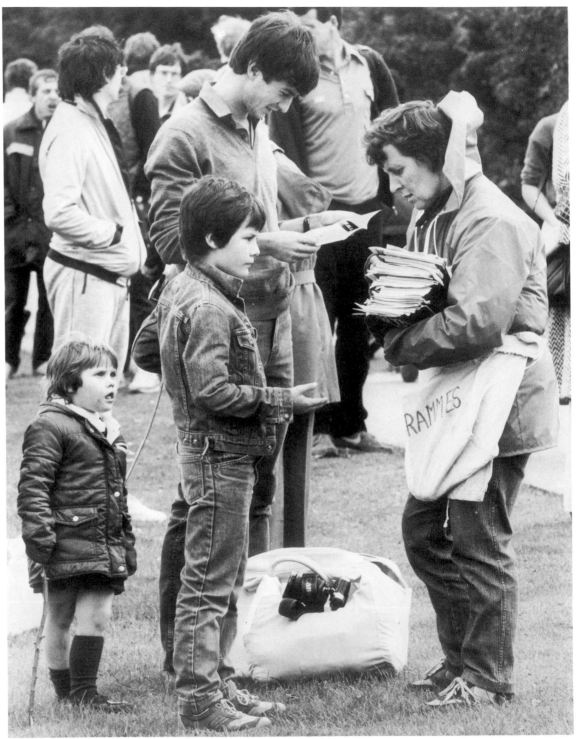

*Buying that essential programme to
see Mum's name is spelt properly.*

Road running clubs. These newer clubs have been set up since the running boom began in the late seventies to cater for the 'citizen' runner who wants to take part in one of Britain's big marathons. Some are affiliated to the WAAA, or to the Women's Cross-country and Road Running Association which governs women's road running. If you join an unaffiliated club you end up paying a 50 pence 'unattached' levy when you enter a race, but that's usually balanced with a cheaper subscription and more informal membership structure. Take care that you don't join a group that's intent on marathon training if you're aiming for more modest targets.

Jogging clubs. What's a jogger? To me, everyone who runs is a runner. Jogging is generally taken to mean running for fitness and fun, usually quite slowly, without any great ambitions, and jogging clubs should welcome those of all abilities who have these modest aims. I know some members of 'jogging' clubs who can run the marathon in less than 2:30 (men) and 3:00 (women). Some jogging clubs are keener on the marathon than others, though most welcome unambitious beginners. Some are affiliated, many are not.

These are three distinct ideas, but in practice the boundaries are very hazy. In your area, you may have a welcoming athletic club with a beginners' section and a jogging club that's full of fast men. In this case, choose the athletic club.

The ideal arrangement is one where joggers and athletes can exist side by side, so that people showing promise can train on the track with the athletics club; newcomers don't feel unwelcome; and everyone shares the same social facilities.

A Big Sister who is a member of a club can gradually introduce her Little Sister to club life when she thinks she is ready. With some clubs that may be immediately, with others perhaps a few months while the beginner builds up confidence and training.

591 Audrey Jaquest and 594 Gillian Neale
from the Watford Joggers Club

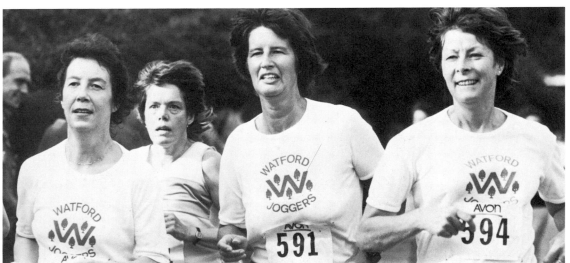

FINDING A CLUB

1. Define your area. How far are you willing to travel to go running? Many clubs meet on Sundays, and so you need to check the reliability of public transport as it might be a problem.

2. Ask at any of the following places:

★   town hall (ask for leisure or recreation department)
★   public library
★   swimming baths
★   leisure centre
★   write to *Running* magazine (address on page 124); enclosing a stamped, self addressed envelope and ask for details of a club in your area
★   call the regional office of the Sports Council (numbers on page 124)
★   if you see some people out running at your sort of pace, ask who they are!

This research may yield two or three names and addresses of running club secretaries in your area. But you still need to do a bit more research.

CHOOSING A CLUB

Now it's time to contact the secretaries and find out if theirs is the right club for you. You need to tell them a bit about yourself, and to ask them some questions to help you decide.

About yourself
★   standard (give a race time or the time of your longest run)
★   age
★   sex (you know you're a woman, but they might not)
★   distance you want to train for
★   do you want to race for the club or just run for fun?

About the club
★   can they help you?
★   how much is membership?
★   what does it include?
★   where and when does the club meet?
★   are there many other people in the club of the same standard as you?
★   can you be put in touch with one of these people?
★   what can you expect on your first run?
★   to what facilities does the club have access? (e.g. changing rooms, bar, track, car park)

First impressions can be lasting impressions, and anyone who is slow to reply to your letter, or sounds off-putting on the phone, may be the secretary of the club you don't want to join. These early researches are time-consuming for you, but they can save you rushing off into the wrong club.

If you are very nervous about going along to the club, why not see if you can arrange to meet some members of the club socially before you go off for your first run? That way, you'll get to know some names and faces, and people in the club can reassure you that they're not going to disappear without you.

STARTING A CLUB

No luck? Is there really no suitable club in your area? Then you must start one! It's easy when you know how. First you need a bit of publicity.

★ local newspapers, especially free ones, are always happy to publicise your efforts. Announce a meeting date and place and just see how many people turn up
★ if you can afford to, print little flyers announcing the meeting, and arrange to put them up in local shops, launderettes, doctors' waiting rooms, pubs, anywhere where people meet
★ tell other people you meet – at the school gates, at the office, at church
★ if you are organising a club from your workplace, put up notices in the tea room, by the photocopier or even in the loo
★ *don't* give a phone number that makes it obvious you're a woman. There are cranks about, and heavy breathers can take all the fun out of running.

Your first meeting

For your first meeting, arrange to meet socially. The needs of the people attending will all be different and trying to organise a bunch of strangers on the run will be difficult, if not impossible. The meeting place doesn't have to be exotic – a pub, someone's house, the office after hours, even a patch of grass in your local park. Ask people to introduce themselves, say what their standards and needs are, and see how they organise themselves.

Find out what people can offer in the way of administrative help. If you like, take a small sub to cover the telephone and postal charges that you will doubtless incur. However enthusiastic you feel at this first meeting this can soon fade if you find you're saddled with all the costs. Delegate from the word go – give everyone a responsibility for some aspect of the group's organisation. But try to keep things informal.

Your second meeting

This is your first *active* meeting together as Maggie's Martyrs, or the Dingle Doddlers or whatever you choose to call yourselves (don't worry if you haven't christened the group at this stage). Someone who accepted a responsibility at the first meeting probably won't be there, while there'll be a few who weren't there last time who will want to be fitted in with your plans. The best thing to do in the early days is to find a natural circuit of about a mile (measure it on a bicycle mileometer or with cotton on a map). Go round a lake or the outside of the park, or twice round the football pitch. Make sure that no-one can complain that they're lost or don't know where they're going.

Warm up together, then make sure all the group run a 'social mile' together at the pace of the slowest. Beginners may well decide that a mile is enough, in which case they should be re-united with warm clothing before everyone runs off again. Someone should stay behind to talk to and encourage beginners. Make sure beginners feel part of the group so that they come back next time and *bring a friend* – that way the club will grow very quickly.

Try to arrange a time trial every month, so that people can measure their progress and see how they match up with others. Some beginners will improve faster than others and will need to change the group they run with; while some faster runners may fall back a group after injury or illness. If there's a social event after the time trial, so much the better – why not organise prizes for the best improvement?

As your group expands you may want to think about facilities like showers and changing rooms – approach your local town hall for advice, or do a deal with a local health, squash or soccer club. But don't worry if you haven't the facilities and your club lives out of car boots – it's not what you've got – it's who you've got.

Opposite: *Anyone can Run Together . . .*

"There was nothing to it really . . ."

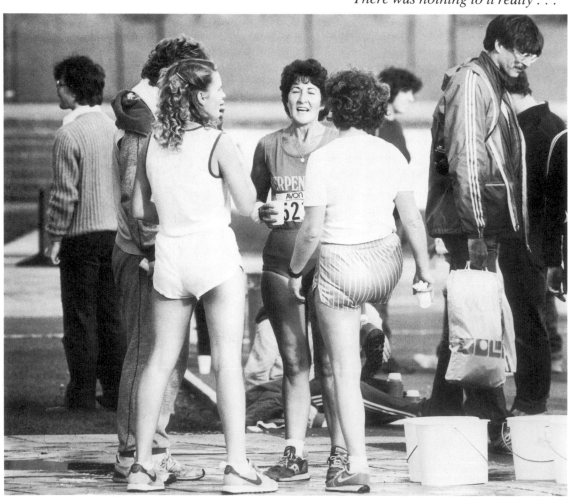

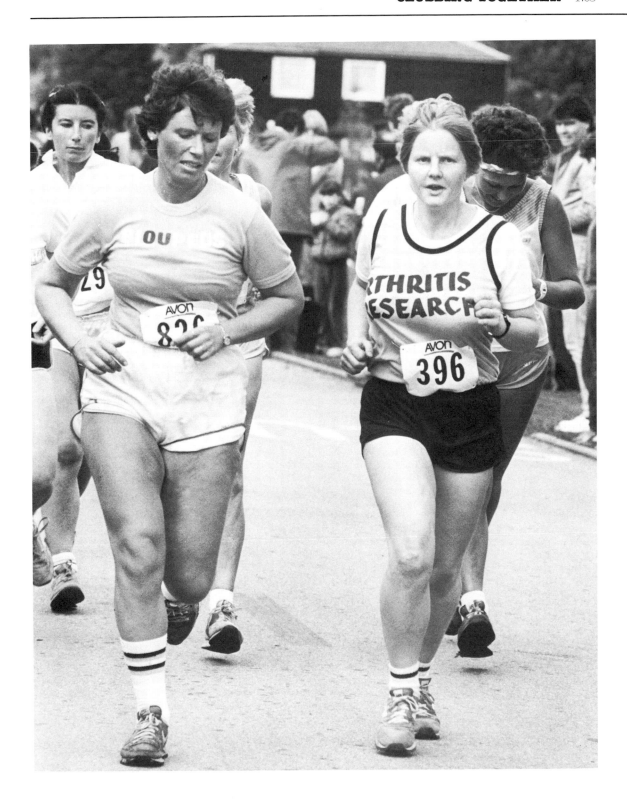

Contacts
Running magazine, 57–61 Mortimer Street, London W1
Sports Council Regional Offices:
North: Durham 49595
North West: 061-834 0338
Yorks/Humberside: Leeds 436443
East Midlands: Nottingham 821887
West Midlands: 021-454 3808
East: Bedford 45222
London/South East: 01-778 8600
South: Reading 595616
South West: Crewkerne 73491
Scotland: 031-225 8411
Wales: Cardiff 397571
Northern Ireland: Belfast 663154
British Orienteering Federation: 41 Dale Road, Matlock, Derbyshire
Fell Runners Association: 165 Penistone Road, Kirkburton, Huddersfield, W. Yorks
British Triathlon Association: 3 Porters Avenue, Dagenham, Essex

CHAPTER ELEVEN
Running for two

When you are pregnant, or trying to conceive, you are easy prey for
all the old wives' tales. Even some very young wives may try and tell
you that women athletes are infertile and all that jogging up and
down is bad for you and the baby.

Sharon Milovsorov, from Wolverhampton, knows all about old wives' tales. 'If I had a
pound for everyone who said, "Should you be running in your condition, dear?" I'd be a
millionaire. But the more comments I had, the more determined I was to show these
people that pregnancy isn't an illness.'

When the Sisters Project started in 1983, Sharon, then 22, wrote offering her services
as a Big Sister. Then she wrote again saying that there was a problem – she was
pregnant. 'No problem,' I said. 'Don't enter for the race, but keep running for as long as
you feel like it, and keep a diary of your progress.' Though every pregnancy is a unique
event, Sharon's diary makes informative reading which she is happy to share with you.

Before she conceived, Sharon was running about 15 miles a week and was just about
to embark on a year's training schedule to run the Wolverhampton Marathon – a
schedule that would take her slowly but surely up to a weekly average of 60 miles a
week. But nature took over. She felt very broody, and she and husband Tony (who's an
international athlete) decided that the time was right to start their family. They didn't
have to wait long.

Months 1–3

The early weeks of Sharon's diary were a dead giveaway. 'So, so, so, tired,' she wrote in
Week 4, 'not worth running.'

'I felt awful this morning' (Week 5), 'so sick I couldn't get out of bed.'

'My boobs hurt when I run' (Week 6).

As if she needed any further evidence, her pregnancy was confirmed in Week 7. 'I am
disappointed,' she said – not about her pregnancy about which she was delighted, but
that 'being fit and healthy I thought I would sail through pregnancy – obviously that is
not the case.' The sickness went into capital letters. 'Felt SO BAD ALL DAY!' she
agonised. But in that week she did manage one run of two miles, taking it very easy –
and she enjoyed it. After the uncertainty of wondering whether or not she was pregnant
she felt more positive about keeping fit.

'I'm glad I've been for at least one run this week. I hope I can keep ticking over till I
feel better.'

Week 8 was very much better – she went out for three two-mile runs and for a swim.
Week 9 was 'disappointing' because the weather was hot and 'the heat never used to
bother me before I was pregnant'.

In Week 10 the old wives' comments started, and with them Sharon's determination to
continue exercising through her pregnancy. 'No wonder so many women let themselves

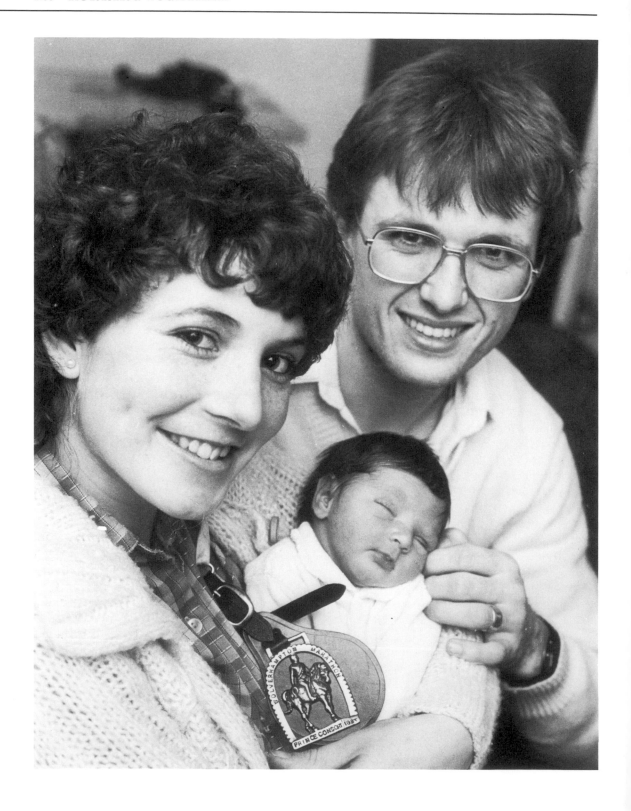

go when they become mothers. They must sit around for nine months then wonder why they get so fat and unfit. NOT ME!'

Thus inspired, she sailed through Week 11 – she ran more, swam faster and added Jane Fonda pregnancy workouts to her schedule.

Months 4–6

As she entered the fourth month of her pregnancy there was encouraging news from Sharon's doctor – first, that she could have a home birth, and second, that as a runner himself, he had no objection to her exercising.

And she started to feel a bit better. In weeks 15 and 16 she went on holiday to Devon. 'No running but plenty of walking – the holiday was just what I needed'; 'I actually feel I'm *blossoming* now!'

Week 18 was a very positive week – she ran twice, swam once and found that it was 'easier to judge my fitness by the swimming'. 'I feel a lot better,' she said, 'and am actually looking forward to the Wolverhampton Marathon 1985!'

The next few weeks were great. The old biddies started to tell Sharon that she was looking well instead of casting doubts on the wisdom of her running. Sharon and Tony got loads of decorating done, she ran four times a week, walked twice a week, swam once, did two Jane Fonda workouts *and* bought herself an exercise bicycle. Phew!

At the end of Week 25 she 'felt excellent. Energy seems to be coming from everywhere. Must be the best week I've had since I've been pregnant.' Pride goes before a fall, though, and the following week she twisted her ankle.

Months 7–9

Now the baby really started to make its presence felt, but Sharon carried on with her exercises – running, cycling, working out, swimming and walking when she felt like it, and putting her feet up when she didn't. 'The baby seems to be pressing on my bladder, and seems very heavy' (Week 27). The women at work were by this time amazed that she was still running. She was fit enough to work an extra month of her pregnancy and go through till Christmas. But the baby felt 'in the way' and the pressure on Sharon's bladder was so much that running was impossible after Week 30. That didn't stop her walking, working out and pedalling mile after mile on the exercise bike, but she did miss the running. 'How I long to take off my "stomach" and go for a really fast sprint down the road,' she said in Week 33.

In Week 35 she walked a total of six miles, cycled eight miles and did three workouts – a 'good week'. But now she was starting to get advice from other mothers which 'doesn't seem to apply to me. I keep expecting things to happen, but I feel so NORMAL. A friend wrote insisting that I take more rest before the baby comes but I don't feel I need to. I don't want to become lazy when I need to be fit for the birth.' Week 35 marked the beginning of her ante-natal classes. 'The exercises seem so easy compared with the workouts.'

Sharon Milovsorov
(Express and Star, Wolverhampton)

In Weeks 36–38, when many mothers are in the armchair snoozing, Sharon averaged 14 miles' walking; four workouts, and six miles on the exercise bike. She had slowed down considerably, and 'really started to feel pregnant' in Week 37.

At the end of Week 39, on 3 February 1984, at 11.15am, Keely Jane Milovsorov was born after a 9½-hour labour with 'no stitches, no gas, no air and no drugs'.

Labour = hard work!

Looking back, Sharon doesn't see how any pregnant woman can do *without* exercise.

'As you become bigger you need to be fit to carry that extra weight around and in nine months' time you need to be at your fittest. Labour is what it says – hard work!

'I took each day as it came, and ran according to how I felt. It's not worth trying to break records or keep up with a training schedule, as you've someone else to think about!

'I was lucky to have a doctor who ran and thought there was nothing wrong with my running. Otherwise I had very few people on my side, and without Tony's encouragement I could so easily have given in.

'A lot of my pregnant friends were ill or tired, had so little energy and couldn't wait to get the thing "over with". I felt so full of energy and stayed an extra five weeks at work. In my pregnant state I felt a lot fitter than the 16- and 17-year-old girls in my office – they said so!

'Of all my friends I had the easiest time. I had no drugs and a wonderful natural birth. The others had pethidine and gas, most screamed through their contractions and all their labours were longer than mine.

'I controlled my contractions fairly easily. Running has helped me learn the importance of relaxed breathing. Having run three marathons I have experienced pain and the desire to give up, but the enjoyment of reaching the finish makes you forget the "bad" miles. Labour is similar in many ways . . . at the start there's a long way to go, and some parts are very tough, giving in is easy, but the finish is a marvellous experience.

'Before having the baby I attended ante-natal classes. I felt I had such a big advantage over the other girls in the class as they only had five lessons of breathing and exercising my body for nine months! Five hours is definitely not enough preparation for labour.

'I went out running when Keely was eight days old. I found the run quite tiring but it was good to be out. My body recovered quickly. But I believe I tried to do too much too soon. I was so eager to get my figure back and get into my jeans that I went mad. I ran and exercised like there was no tomorrow. I also starved myself at mealtimes which was totally wrong. As a result, my milk dried up. When Keely was six weeks I had mastitis and was told to give up breastfeeding. I was so upset and felt annoyed at putting myself first. Next time it will be different.

'Keely is a good and happy baby and I'm sure it's because I'm happy and relaxed with her. My running has taken on a new meaning. I've had more ambitions for myself – I want to enter more races, I want to be the slimmest mother at the school gates, and most of all when Keely's older I want her to be proud of me and for people to think we're sisters! I feel with running I can achieve all these and more.'

Sharon was sensible in her pregnancy, and followed the golden rules we looked at earlier – to run when you're up, and rest when you're down. As a nursing mother she wasn't so clever – but she won't make that mistake again, and others can learn from it.

Mary Swindles, from North Harrow, was 30, and eight months into her third pregnancy when she joined the Sisters Project. She had done very little running since. Her husband Gordon is also a runner and, says Mary, 'I was selfish enough to resent him running while I couldn't when I was pregnant.' The Project was an incentive for Mary to think about her body and to do something about it after Andrew was born at the end of May 1983.

Mary breastfed Andrew successfully for eight months before he was weaned. Like Sharon, she was impatient to get back into shape – and her running shorts – but her healthy appetite and her experience made sure that she ate enough both to nurse Andrew and get back to running. She started running six days after the birth, when she went out for a six-minute jog. Four months later she completed the Avon 10 in 82 minutes. The following year she ran it in 72 minutes – faster than she'd ever run before she had Andrew.

Spence Ingerson, 34, from West London, also joined the Project to motivate herself back into shape after her baby daughter was born in January. Spence says she was 'lucky'. 'I jogged right up to the last few days. I walked to the hospital – although I was trying to jog, it was too painful – I did not know that I was in pre-labour. The results? Steady blood pressure, high haemoglobin count (even just after birth), rapid recovery. I had a short [four-hour] but fierce labour which was much harder than my 3:30 marathon. I could do sit-ups within the week and the 25 pounds I had gained was off again within two months.

'But I stress – I was lucky. Each woman is different and it is depressing to read in running books that so-and-so ran three hours before birth. For some women it is just *too* painful.'

The message here is loud and clear: *Every woman, every pregnancy, is different.* The experiences of these three women were all different and you should not try to compare yourself or compete with others.

Expert advice

When it comes down to it *you* are the expert. You know what your body is capable of – you know when to push it and when to relax. But at this important time of your life – and your baby's life – there are still many questions you want answered – questions that your doctor may not have time to answer; or that s/he will dodge. I put some of your questions to Dr Beverley Kane.

Will running affect my chances of conceiving?

There's little to worry about here. It's true that many top women athletes don't menstruate, and when you start to run you may also find that your menstrual cycle changes in some way. Your periods may become irregular or cease altogether. That may be good news if it means less monthly discomfort for you, but it can be worrying if you are hoping to conceive. It's widely believed (but not proven) that weight loss is responsible for the absence of ovulation and menstruation, but many women find that their regular cycle returns without a gain in weight. If your cycle is disrupted, and this worries you, you should look for other explanations as well. For example, have you been overdoing things at work? Or travelling a lot? Have you moved house or had a death in the family?

In Chapter Seven, we looked at the importance of keeping a diary recording the changes in your daily routine, your feelings, your menstrual cycle and any other regular patterns you notice in your life. If you are very concerned about your irregular cycle you should try and highlight some relevant patterns in your diary and ask your GP to refer you to a specialist. Your diary could provide some valuable information for the specialist.

If you are not ovulating, it's generally true to say that you won't conceive, but don't bank on it! Ovulation can return at any time, especially a time of relaxation like a holiday, an enforced lay-off through injury or missing a couple of contraceptive pills – even sex itself can trigger the system back into action! If you make love during this time you could well become pregnant before your next period – but how will you know? This is what happened to top marathoner Ingrid Kristiansen who was nearly five months pregnant before she started to wonder why she wasn't running so well. She hadn't menstruated for some time, so she didn't have one of the first warning signs of pregnancy – a missed period.

If I run in pregnancy, am I more likely to miscarry?

No. About one in six pregnancies ends in miscarriage, but there is no evidence that women who exercise in pregnancy are more likely to miscarry. A healthy foetus takes a strong hold in the womb and gentle, rhythmic exercise like running cannot dislodge it. A shock, like falling downstairs or crashing the car, is different – in this case you will need careful observation to make sure that everything is all right.

An unhealthy embryo, which is the result of incomplete cell division or has a chromosomal abnormality, will miscarry regardless of the exercise you do or don't do – this is nature's way of protecting you from having abnormal babies.

You should be prepared to give up running if you have miscarried before because of a weak or 'incompetent' cervix, where the baby develops normally but you are unable to carry it. In this case the doctor may insist that you rest between the third and fifth months, if not longer, to increase your chances of keeping the baby, and you will probably be encouraged to have a stitch to hold the cervix closed until nearer the date of delivery.

It's very important to think positively if things go wrong. Words like 'incompetent' and 'spontaneous abortion' (simply another term for miscarriage) do nothing for a woman's morale at a difficult time in her life. Don't take them personally, but do everything you can to find out how you can prevent miscarrying a second time.

Sue Fletcher of Welwyn conceived shortly after the Avon 10 in October 1983, but lost her baby the following February. She had already miscarried once before due to a weak cervix, so she was wise to take her doctor's advice and not to run during her pregnancy. She had a suture to try and remedy the weak cervix, but miscarried anyway. Thinking positively about herself, she went off on a skiing holiday, and then started running again. Though at the time of writing she had not conceived again, she did not blame running in any way for her difficulties either in conceiving or carrying. Neither did her doctors, though naturally a few 'old wives' had something to say about it.

What warning signs should I look out for?

The same signs as any other pregnant woman. A *rise in blood pressure* can cause concern. Your GP or ante-natal clinic will monitor your blood pressure and may admit you to hospital if they have any doubts. The worst thing you can do if this happens is worry – about your job or your family or whether the baby will be all right. The best thing you can do is put your feet up and *relax*.

Don't ignore *bleeding*, however little. 'Spotting' may be the first signs of a miscarriage which you can avoid. Don't wait till it's too late because you don't want to bother the doctor!

You will doubtless suffer the uncomfortable swelling that comes with water retention (similar to the bloated pre-menstrual feeling) but if in the later months of your pregnancy the swelling gets worse and affects your hands and face, and is accompanied by a weight gain of more than one pound per week, you will probably need more frequent pre-natal checks. You should also not exercise if, after 20 weeks, your blood pressure suddenly goes up.

Can running help stave off morning sickness?

Sorry, there's no evidence to suggest that it can, as Sharon found to her disappointment. Like period pains, some women find that running helps, while others just don't want to know. Reassure yourself that it's a problem suffered by millions of women and that you'll feel better by the fourth month. I know many other women besides Sharon who say that the best time for running is between months four and six – when you are less worried and more relaxed about yourself, but haven't started to get really big. So even if you don't run much in months one to three, do have another go a bit later on.

The favourite remedies may just work for you: eating little and often; munching dry toast or water biscuits before you get up in the morning; extra vitamin B_6.

What should I eat, and how much weight should I expect to put on?

Stick with the balanced, fresh diet we looked at in Chapter Seven, making sure that you eat plenty of iron (particularly in liver and green leafy vegetables) and calcium (put milk and cheese on to your 'eat more' list (page 93) but choose low fat varieties). Try to drink four glasses of skimmed milk a day. You should also drink about eight glasses of water a day. Limit the amount of tea and coffee you drink.

I don't think you need me to tell you to leave off alcohol and cigarettes. The media will tell you, your own doctor will tell you, and most important, if you listen closely your body will also tell you what's right and what's wrong. You will lose your taste for certain things and develop tastes for others. If you get a craving for something like chocolate, indulge it – but only if it makes you feel better! The average weight gain in pregnancy is 25 lb – but this depends on your height and build.

How much running should I do, and how fast?

You should do *just as much running as you feel like*. No doctor or coach can predict how you will feel or behave, and no-one should push you beyond limits you can't achieve. You shouldn't race, or use speedwork in your training. Think about it: any exercise which leaves you breathless can also leave the baby short of breath. You probably won't want to race anyway. Aggression and competitive urges seem to float away when you are pregnant so that you automatically slow down.

As a rough guide, you should not exercise above 70 per cent of your maximum heart rate (page 74). Take your pulse immediately after your run. If you are 20 years, it should not be higher than 140 beats a minute; if you are 30, 133 beats a minute; if you are 40, 126 beats a minute.

If you are already fit – and you have completed the first 20 weeks in Chapter Eight, then aim simply to maintain the level of running you did before you were pregnant, but without worrying about the pace. Don't worry if you don't manage this. Thirty to forty minutes three times a week is quite enough.

If you are unfit, but it's early in your pregnancy, and you have carefully read through the early part of this book, there's nothing to stop you from starting running, very gently – five minutes, three times a week. If you feel like it, add half a minute to each run the following week so that you run three × 5½ mins; then three × 6 mins. As with the building blocks in Chapter Eight, you should only progress if you can honestly say that each week has been as good as, or better than, the previous week.

My friend could run five miles when she was seven months pregnant. I can't. Yet we used to train together at the same pace.
As we said earlier, you shouldn't try and compare yourself with other women, or even compare your own pregnancies. You must go by how you feel, not by what others have done.

What other exercises should I do?
Again, it's up to you. Sharon sensibly built up a balanced programme of exercise – running, swimming, cycling, workouts from the Jane Fonda pregnancy book, and walking. In the later stages when it was too uncomfortable to run she had the other forms of exercise to fall back on, and was able to walk a mile the day before Keely was born.

Slow stretching and yoga are particularly recommended, especially later on in pregnancy when the spine starts to curve under the weight of the baby. Take advantage of the ante-natal classes on offer, but don't just rely on them to keep you fit for a long labour!

And if you can't run, don't hang up your running shoes. They will probably be more comfortable than any of your other shoes as you get bigger!

I can't hold my water. Help!
Nearly all pregnant women feel the need to go to the loo all the time, especially as the pregnancy progresses. If you really can't hold it in, try wearing a sanitary towel. A tampon inserted into the vagina will press against the urethra (the neighbouring tube through which the urine passes) and is recommended as an effective remedy for 'the dribbles'.

And try Kegel exercises which strengthen the group of muscles known as the pelvic floor muscles. These muscles start and stop the flow of urine, and contract uncontrollably when you have an orgasm. Exercising them can help control incontinence, make sex more enjoyable, and strengthen the muscles for childbirth. Exercise them by contracting hard for a second and then releasing. Do this 10 times. Once you have found where the muscles are, you can repeat the exercise several times during the day, wherever you are (no-one can see!). Also make sure that you have regular urine tests throughout your pregnancy in case your incontinence is linked with an infection.

Will I have a shorter labour than an unfit woman?

Not necessarily, but as a fit woman you will definitely be able to cope better with labour. There's no evidence to suggest, either, that runners have fewer complications, or higher birthweight babies, or that their babies are more likely to be born on time. As we said before, every pregnancy is different.

When can I start running again after my baby is born?

Don't assume that, like Ingrid Kristiansen, you can be up and about and ready for a marathon in four months' time. But *do* start thinking positively about getting back into shape through exercise. Start walking as soon as you feel like it after delivery, and start running when bleeding has stopped and your stitches (if you had them) have healed comfortably. Go back over the Building Blocks in Chapter Eight and build up slowly. Take advantage of the post-natal exercises offered by your doctor or clinic.

Should I run if I am breastfeeding?

There's no evidence to suggest that *exercise* decreases milk production. What is more common is that, as in Sharon's case, in your efforts to restore your figure you will start cutting back on essential items in your diet when in fact you need to eat even *more* than you did when you were pregnant. Nursing, as she found, *isn't* the time for a reducing diet! The discomfort of large, nursing breasts will slow you down, so it's best to run just after a feed.

Will motherhood make me a better runner?

Sharon and Mary are now running faster times than before, but no, there's no guarantee that pregnancy will make you faster. However, many women use pregnancy as a time to change their lifestyles for the better. They change their diet, they give up smoking, and ease off the pressure at work. They claim they are doing it 'for the baby' – which is a good excuse to be doing it for themselves. As they plan their new routine they can make sure they have the time to run – and often their running improves! Positive changes made in pregnancy can last you the rest of your life.

Contraception

On average, we are fertile for 35 years each, and most of us spend a large part of that time trying *not* to become pregnant. I'm often asked if there is a 'best' contraceptive for runners. There isn't. There is no one method that suits every woman in every age group.

You shouldn't be afraid of Family Planning Clinics. You may wait a long time, but you usually get a good deal – regular blood pressure checks, cervical smears (but remember to chase up the results), and breast examination and a chance to ask questions and get sensible advice, which your own GP may not always have time to dispense.

Let's look now at the most popular forms of contraception, and how they affect the active woman.

The pill (used by over three million women in the UK)

The long-term effects of taking the contraceptive pill – either the combination or mini (progesterone only) pill – are still not known. Despite the horror stories in the press, millions of women happily take the pill till their mid-thirties or even longer without any side effects or problems. They are liberated by its reliability, having lighter periods as well as being able to manipulate their periods around important events in their lives.

But many active, health-conscious women are beginning to question the wisdom of a daily dose of synthetic hormones, to protect them on the relatively few days every month when they are fertile. Women coming off the pill after many years of continuous use often feel clearer-headed; they may lose weight even if they didn't gain it in the first place; and they feel more in touch with the natural rhythms of their bodies.

Research at Salford University indicates that the pill can slow you down! These studies have only, as yet, been carried out on a handful of athletes for a short period of time – but it's food for thought. Effectiveness: 100 per cent (combined), 98 per cent (mini).

IUD (UK current use 912,000)

The intrauterine device (IUD) is an ideal birth control method for women who have had children and do not have heavy periods. It has not been as successful on childless women. There are more exaggerated stories surrounding this device than any other – perforations of the womb, pregnancies with the IUD still in place, or ectopic pregnancies where the fertilised egg implants not in the womb but in the Fallopian tube. The statistics are small, but gruesome to ponder. And if you are becoming interested in your body and how it works, the idea of a 'foreign body' anchored in your womb may turn you right off.

It doesn't? Then you're lucky, and this may well be your ideal method. Can an IUD 'fall out' when you're running? No, unless it is going to anyway. Check the strings regularly. Effectiveness: 96–98 per cent.

Barrier methods (UK use 1,824,000)

Used properly, the diaphragm and sheath can be very effective. The attraction is that you only use them when you need them, and they don't cause major bodily changes. The turn-off comes when you have to interrupt the passionate scenes to organise yourselves – you need to be, and have, a very understanding partner.

The effectiveness of both methods is increased when you also use spermicide – often evil-smelling cream, gel, pessaries or foam which can irritate some women – and some men, too. But unlike the pill, these chemicals are only in contact with a small area of the body and will not affect your moods or your menstrual cycle.

Like the IUD, a properly fitted diaphragm cannot 'fall out' when you run. But there are two things which your doctor or family planning adviser should tell you. One is that you shouldn't sink into a bath within six hours of your last intercourse, and so dilute the effect of the spermicide. If you make love and run in the morning, this can make life difficult. The other is that if you lose more than half a stone, as you may well do when you start exercising, you should go back to the doctor who fitted your diaphragm to make sure it still fits. Effectiveness: 97 per cent with spermicide and careful use.

Natural methods (UK use 570,000)

There was a time when the only method of birth control open to Roman Catholics and other people with strong moral or religious beliefs was the 'calendar' method, often called 'Vatican Roulette' as an indication of its unreliability! This was only of use to women with very regular menstrual cycles who could calculate their fertile times very accurately.

But times have changed, and there are other ways of monitoring your fertile life – either to prevent pregnancy or to make sure of it. These ways are fast finding favour with women who like their bodies and aren't squeamish about them; and who are in steady relationships with understanding men. If, after reading Chapter Seven, you prove to be a good diarist, you are well on the way to skilful birth control by natural methods.

The length of your menstrual cycle may not be constant, but there are two regular events in the cycle which you can chart to assess the fertile days of the month. On these days you either use a barrier method of contraception or not have full sexual intercourse.

Just before you ovulate every month, your temperature drops. After ovulation it rises noticeably and stays that way until your next period. Taking your temperature daily can tell you the safe days after you ovulate. It won't necessarily tell you which are the safe days before you ovulate, although familiarity with the method and your usual cycle length may, in time, help you determine when those days are.

The Billings method, developed by two Australian doctors, relies on changes in the mucus secreted by the cervix. By examining the mucus every day, and recording what you see, you can pinpoint the fertile days in your cycle. To some of you this may sound worse than blowing your nose and then examining your handkerchief, but it really is very simple to understand with practice – and works both ways, for you can also establish the best time to make love if you are hoping to conceive. Effectiveness: 83–93 per cent with careful use.

Sterilisation/vasectomy (used by over 200,000 couples in UK)
These are irreversible decisions, and it is often difficult to obtain a doctor's consent to a sterilisation or vasectomy operation if you have no children. Weigh up all the advantages and disadvantages carefully. Sterilisation may make you brighter and more confident in your life and your running – or you can sink into a depression that part of your life is over. You will also need time off running to have the operation and recover from it. Effectiveness: 1 in 1,000 vasectomies and 1 in 500 sterilisations fail as a contraceptive.

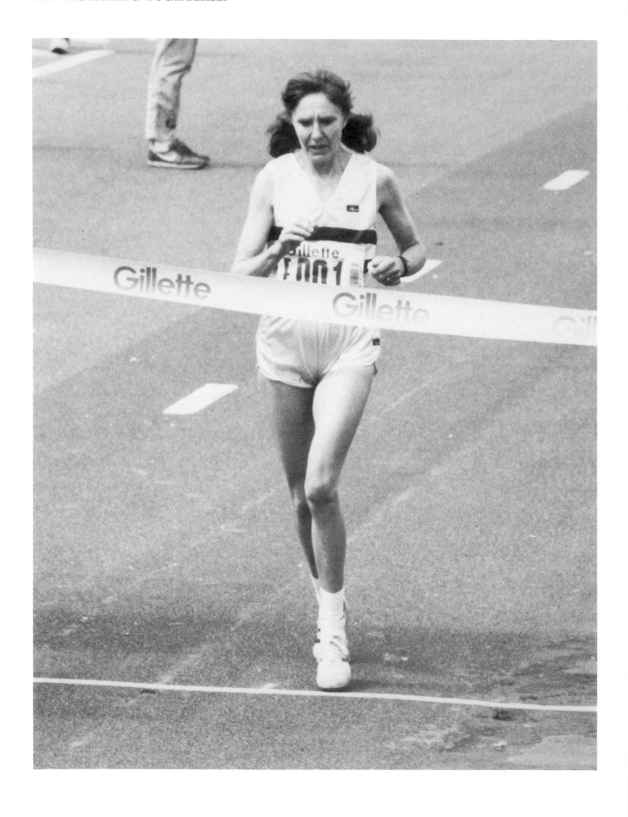

CHAPTER TWELVE
Life after 50

In the first *Sunday Times* National Fun Run in 1978, there were 43 women listed as 50–59 – none at all aged 60–70. In 1981, Madge Sharples became a star in the first London Marathon because it was so unusual for a woman over 60 to be doing such a thing. But now the veteran ranks are swelling, and the competition for age-related prizes is becoming tougher! In 1984, in the sixth *Sunday Times* Fun Run, there were 151 women between 50–59 years; 22 60–69 and six over-70s.

What attractions does running hold for the older woman? Is it really the fount of eternal youth?

The menopause can be a very negative experience (I'm getting old . . . I'm past my best . . . I'm not attractive any more . . . my body's shrinking). Women trapped by their bodies cannot cope with hot flushes, night sweats, and the emotional switchback which the change of life brings. After the uncertainty of childbearing years, for some women the menopause is a change for the better – and women of this age have a freedom and independence that their younger sisters envy.

How you change your life is up to you. As runners, we are aware of our bodies and the way they move and change – and we learn to adapt positively to those changes. We aren't trapped by our bodies but actually quite like them – in short, we are equipped to think positively about the menopause.

Joyce Smith, of Wimbledon, is 56 (not to be confused with Joyce Smith the 47-year-old international!). Joyce started running in 1980, and her 'change' has definitely been one for the better.

'My image of myself has changed,' she says. 'I've liked myself these last couple of years more than I've ever done before. I didn't have a good opinion of myself before running. I thought of myself as a dull, dowdy middle-aged woman with an ugly body. I have positive feelings about myself now.'

What exactly happens at the menopause? When we are born, our ovaries have a limited number of ova (eggs) available for fertilisation. During our fertile years we release one of these every month (ovulation). Later, as supplies run out, the egg release becomes more erratic. Sometimes we ovulate, sometimes we do not; sometimes we menstruate, sometimes we do not; and our once predictable hormones are thrown off balance so that sometimes we feel fine, sometimes we feel as if we have pre-menstrual tension all month!

Hot flushes, night sweating and vaginal dryness are the classic signs of the menopause though severe symptoms are the exception, not the rule. All are connected with low levels of oestrogen which, when you are menstruating normally, is in regular supply.

Joyce Smith (All Sport)

Of more importance to active women is the fact that oestrogen plays an important part in maintaining the body's use of calcium, protein and Vitamin D – all vital in bone growth. When the oestrogen level drops, the bones start to waste away very slowly. This is why old women so easily suffer broken bones, and why they 'shrink' and become hump-backed as the spine shortens.

This condition is known as *osteoporosis*. The good news is that regular exercise and a balanced diet can help prevent osteoporosis. Research has shown that the bones of active people are stronger.

But if the weakening process has already begun, you are more likely to become injured if you take up running. There is also research that suggests that women (of all ages) who do not menstruate are deficient in oestrogen and thus run the risk of osteoporosis. Women at risk should take up exercise more gradually and mix running with other aerobic sports like swimming and cycling which don't put so much weight on the legs.

Hormone Replacement Therapy (HRT) tops up the oestrogen levels in menopausal women who then do not suffer hot flushes, night sweats, vaginal dryness and osteoporosis. Like the contraceptive pill, HRT is a controversial treatment. Some people swear that it has enriched their lives; others say that it isn't natural. In fact, the treatment is more natural than the Pill in that the oestrogen usually comes from natural sources, rather than being made up in the laboratory. The long-term effects of HRT, like the pill, aren't yet established.

Supporters of HRT say that the risks of cancer of the womb or breast, stroke and heart disease are less in women taking the treatment, while others in the medical profession are adamant that the treatment *increases* the risk of cancer of the womb. If HRT makes you feel better, and enriches your life, you may want to gamble with these risks anyway, on the grounds that you have nothing to lose.

Brenda Green swears by HRT. She is 55 and started the treatment when she was 48. Every six months, Brenda has a small 'implant' inserted in her abdomen under local anaesthetic. The advantage of an implant is that it by-passes the digestive system. At the same time she has her blood pressure monitored, a blood sample taken, and a probe to establish whether there are cancerous cells in the lining of the womb. She is also asked to examine her breasts for lumps and report on any unusual bleeding – but so far there have been no warning signs.

The benefits? Brenda simply doesn't look 55. When she compares her lifestyle with other women of her age, she is amazed at how young she feels. She has none of the mood swings, hot flushes, or dryness. The treatment has enhanced her family and social life. 'Some people say it isn't natural,' she says, 'but I wouldn't have it any other way.'

Not having known any other way, Brenda doesn't know whether running, which she started in 1982, would have relieved some of the symptoms of the menopause. Hilary Brindley, 52, from South London, has been running since 1976, and having used the pill for some years is unwilling to 'mess around with nature again'. Hilary is sure that running helped her to cope with the symptoms of the menopause which, for her, are mild, and haven't interfered with her life. There are many other women who say that running has helped them cope with this difficult time of life.

Brenda Green

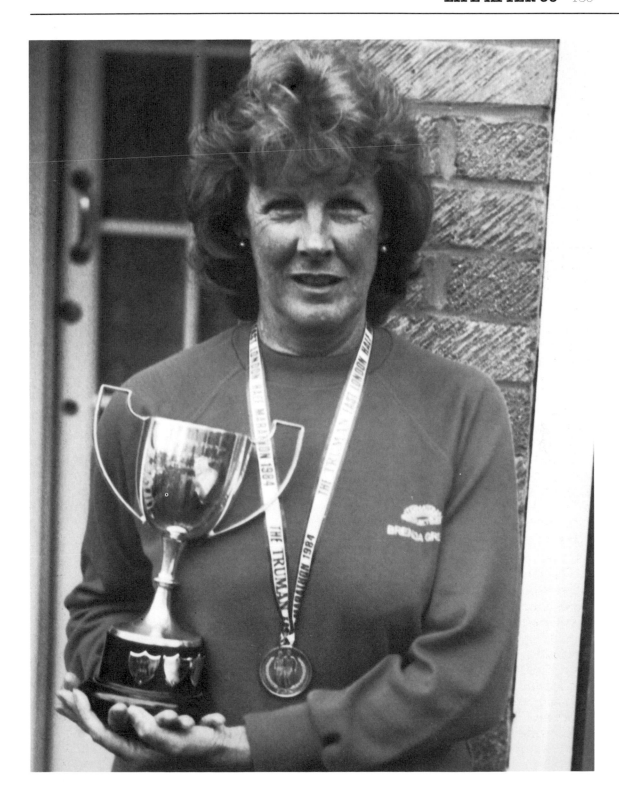

One of them is Mary Harrison (51) of Wootton Bassett. Running has helped her – she's sure that *coffee* is to blame for hot flushes!

Kath Brandwood, 48, of Twickenham, was badly hit by the menopause, and felt she would like to look into HRT, if her GP were sympathetic, which she wasn't. Kath's certain that her problems would be 10 times worse if she didn't run. 'I'm too busy running, swimming and looking after Little Sisters to give it a thought some days.'

The menopause seems to hit some women harder than others. Many women have no symptoms at all. Others can 'run off' the symptoms without further treatment, especially if their diet is healthy and balanced and contains plenty of calcium (from milk products or supplements prescribed by the doctor). But it pays to be cautious, and never to increase your training too quickly – any injury you sustain may take longer to repair than a younger woman's.

Hysterectomy

The menopause is a difficult stage in every woman's life. An unlucky few have to have their wombs removed surgically (hysterectomy) because they are cancerous, or bleeding too heavily. Unlike the menopause, a hysterectomy is a sudden end to a woman's fertile years. It can be very depressing. Can running help?

Yes, says Joan Roberts of Hyde, who had a hysterectomy when she was 42. Before that she had very heavy periods, caused by fibroids (non-cancerous lumps in the womb). Joan started running a year after the operation.

'I felt that the hysterectomy had spoiled my figure – I had a very flabby tum. Running got me back into shape, made me feel good, and took away the feeling that part of my life was over. My depression was so severe at times that I felt suicidal and didn't want to go on. Running lifted me out of that, too.'

Joan's operation did not involve removal of the ovaries, so she later developed all the symptoms of the menopause – but running 'seems to control the hot flushes'.

Retirement

It seems crazy to me that on her sixtieth birthday a working woman is suddenly expected to sever all her connections with her working life, and be put out to grass. It is no wonder that retirement leaves a hole in a woman's life. For some it is the beginning of the end. They feel they have outlived their usefulness. They stop seeing their friends. They don't need a gold watch or a teamaker to announce the passage of time. It just slips from their grasp.

Pauline Frew wrote at the beginning of the Sisters Project: 'I am 62 years of age and for that reason imagine I shall be of no use to you.' How wrong she was. Pauline was about to retire after an active teaching career. A few years earlier she had broken her arm badly and was unable to carry on playing badminton with her husband John.

'I missed the exercise and put on weight, which did nothing for my morale.' She ran the *Sunday Times* Fun Run in 1982, but needed the Sisters Project to encourage her to run further. She started the Avon 10 training schedule, but then went to her doctor to have her blood pressure taken for our records. At 185/90 he pronounced it too high and forbade her to run for three weeks.

'I have a suspicion,' she said, 'that the doctor thinks I should do "something more suitable for my age" but the last thing I want to do, apart from killing myself off – is to give up running. I recover very quickly from a run and feel far fitter when I am running than when I am not.' By the end of the five-month training period her blood pressure was down to a more sedate 160/85.

Now, she says, 'I am without doubt fitter and more energetic and purposeful when I am running regularly and I cease to dwell on the fact that my teaching days are over. There is no scope for brooding over days gone by. I never cease to be amazed in races at the way youngsters accept me as another competitor and show no surprise at my age. The age gap loses its significance when you are all struggling up the same hill . . .'

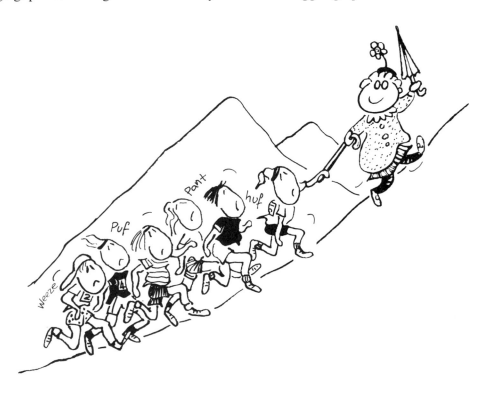

CHAPTER THIRTEEN
Looking the part

'If you get worried by people shouting remarks as you run,' says
Fiona Nixon, of Tonypandy, 'it's worth buying professional looking
kit. People aren't so rude if they think you're a good athlete!' Sally
Justice of Clapham agrees: 'You don't run well if you don't feel right.'

Good supportive and cushioning running shoes are the most important item in your
wardrobe, as we found in Chapter Five. Up till now, I've suggested that you get by with
any old baggy clothes. But now you're not so old and baggy! As you change shape and
become more confident, you may well want to buy the clothes that go with your new
body and that make you look the part.

   There's a confusing range of running clothing on the market. What do you need and
what can you do without? What are you meant to wear for what? I've devised a basic kit
for you for winter and summer. For gear specially for running, go back to that good shop
that sold you your running shoes – for other clothes the world, or at least the High
Street, is your oyster. Remember Bunty's wardrobe? Well, now she's grown up and
started to run . . .

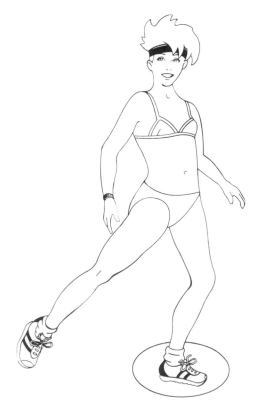

Bunty – the Adult Version

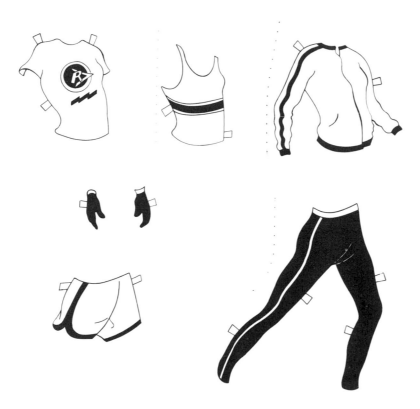

Bunty's running outfit

Basics

Bras. Lucky the woman who is small-breasted, and doesn't knock herself out at every stride. If this is you, you may be able to run quite happily without a bra, as long as your nipples don't chafe against your T-shirt or vest. 'Jogger's nipple', where the nipples do chafe against the clothing and may even bleed, is a bit of a joke among non-runners, who assume that it is a feminine complaint – but usually women are more sensible, and wearing a good bra reduces the risk of chafing. If you run bra-less you can prevent friction either by rubbing petroleum jelly on your nipples or by taping sticking plaster over them.

If you do need a bra to run in, make sure that it:
★   is stretchy enough to move with you, but not so stretchy that it still lets your breasts wobble up and down
★   has cups of absorbent material which are either seamless or have well-finished seams
★   doesn't have trimmings, fastenings or bindings which are likely to chafe
★   has no wires
★   has a broad band under the bust which makes sure the bra doesn't ride up

Your favourite chain store bra may meet these needs, in which case it isn't worth shelling out extra money for a special sports bra. I wear sports bras all the time because they're so comfortable. They are usually available in sizes up to 40D. They either come in conventional style with back fastening and adjustable straps, or a style that has no fastenings and pulls over your head. This style reduces the risk of chafing, but if your breast size changes for any reason (you might lose weight as your training progresses or you might swell up due to pre-menstrual water retention) you cannot make adjustments. Diana Mealing of Bristol doesn't favour this type.

'I don't like pulling it over my head when it rolls in sausages around my sweaty skin!'

Maureen Farish, of Bromley, used to wear a sports bra 'till I saw myself on the TV coverage of the 1982 London Marathon. The awful sight of my breasts bobbing up and down independently gave me a real fright!' Maureen now prefers a cross-over bra which she finds supportive and *not* bouncy.

Carol Garnett of Cramlington tried to make do with an ordinary bra, but ran into problems. 'My breasts became extremely lumpy. My GP said it was fibrosis of both breasts caused by not wearing a correct supporting bra while running. I had to bind myself with bandages for a few weeks after that.' Since wearing a sports bra, the problem hasn't recurred.

Unless you are very confident of your sizing, it's best to try before you buy. If you go to the corsetry section of a large department store, you can try on a number of makes and sizes. Jump up and down in the bra. If your breasts bounce uncomfortably, then the bra isn't suitable for running.

More running shops are stocking sports bras now, and providing the facilities to try them on privately. About time. When I was first buying them it was a hit-and-miss affair – I had to go round behind the shoe boxes and hope that one of the male shop assistants wouldn't need to go into the stockroom!

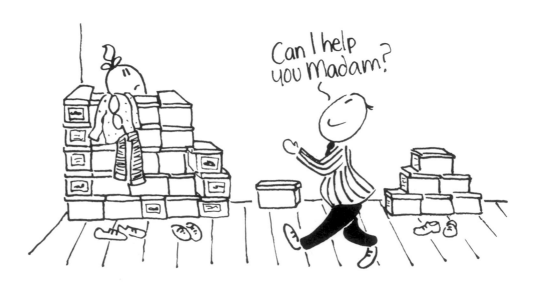

Knickers. Snug, absorbent cotton briefs are best, as nylon can aggravate vaginal infections like thrush. Some nylon shorts have a cotton-lined gusset. You can wear these with or without knickers underneath, as you can the snug-fitting towelling shorts favoured by track runners.

Socks. Socks fill in the spaces between your feet and your running shoes and cut down the friction between shoe and foot which causes blisters. There are special sports socks on the market, but any sock will do if it is non-chafing (bad seams across the toenails can cause blackness or lifting); long-lasting; absorbent; and washable. Cushioning is an additional luxury – loops inside the sock under the sole of the foot make the socks more comfortable and absorbent. Don't fight shy of synthetic materials – they are cheaper and longer-lasting, more easily washable than cotton and wool, and surprisingly cool in hot weather.

Clean dry socks mean fewer blisters. If you skin is sensitive to detergent, wash the socks in soap and make sure they are thoroughly rinsed before drying.

Summer clothes

Shorts. Horrified by the thought of wearing shorts in public? Take heart from Judy Wurr:

'Wear shorts whatever your legs are like. I'm known locally as "thunder thighs" but I don't care – at least I can run.'

You have a choice of material and style here. Track runners favour cotton towelling briefs, but these top athletes are usually blessed with small bottoms and don't have to endure abuse from lorry drivers. Choose these briefs only if you find them comfortable and flattering.

The most popular shorts with road runners are made of lightweight nylon, usually with a built-in brief that may or may not be cotton-lined. These are more flattering for bigger bottoms, and though they cover more of you up, they don't restrict free movement. They also come in some lovely colours. They can be expensive, but they are nice enough to wear on holiday or around the house on a hot day. They wash and dry very quickly.

Always try shorts on in the shop. If the shorts look big enough, the inner pant, if there is one, may not be. Raise your leg so that your thigh is parallel with the floor. If the shorts are not comfortable over your widest range of movements, buy the next size up. Your stride may be no more than a shuffle now, but you don't want to feel that your legs are tied together when you start to pick up speed.

Look out for well-finished seams and a soft waistband (the more lines of stitching the better). A trim round the hem of the shorts may look smart, but make sure it won't chafe the legs uncomfortably.

T-shirts. You can never have enough loose-fitting, plain cotton T-shirts, either to wear while running or to put on over a vest after your run. There's no need to spend much money. Some races give free T-shirts to all finishers; or you can buy them in Oxfam shops or at jumble sales. Cut off the neckband and/or sleeves if they are too tight, or cut the shape of a vest, making sure that the armholes aren't too big. Don't hem it, but leave the edges unfinished.

Vests. If you're happy with a T-shirt, fine. But for hot weather training and racing it's nice to have a lightweight nylon vest which absorbs sweat and takes it away from the body. Nylon dries much more quickly than cotton. Many running vests are made with a mesh panel which allows sweat to evaporate even more quickly, and thus keep you cool on a hot day. You can usually get a vest that matches or co-ordinates with your shorts.

Try a vest on with the bra and shorts you'll be wearing it with and make sure that they all agree with each other and there aren't vast areas of bra or midriff showing. Make sure that the armholes are not too tight, but not so loose that most of your bra shows. Some vests have little tabs to hold the bra strap under the shoulder of the vest – but if not you can improvise with a safety pin or sew in little tabs which fasten with a press-stud. As with all your running clothes, look out for well-finished seams and bindings.

Sunhat. A cheap cotton sunhat or cap is essential in very hot sunshine. Believe it or not, a cabbage leaf inside your hat will absorb the sun's rays and help prevent sunstroke.

Winter clothes
Thermal top. Whatever else you buy for winter, you should invest in a long-sleeved 'thermal' top. Thermal clothing is made from tightly knit synthetic fibres which trap body heat but allow sweat to evaporate – unlike cotton, which hangs damp and heavy on the skin, and can cool you down dramatically if you slow down or the wind speeds up. It washes easily and quickly and will be dry in time for your next run. Don't tumble dry or iron. You can wear anything – vest, T-shirt, sweatshirt, rainjacket on top of this important layer.

Sweatshirts. As for T-shirts, you can never have enough fleecy lined sweatshirts – for running in over your thermal vest, to put on afterwards (in more than one layer if necessary) or lightly looped around your waist on those spring and autumn days when it might get chilly halfway through your run. Have at least one hooded sweatshirt in your collection. Again, look out for second-hands and giveaways.

Tights. Keeping your legs warm is particularly important if you are a newer, slower runner, when on winter days you will take a long time to warm up and then, if you slow down, you can cool rapidly. Cold legs are more likely to get stiff and injured. You can choose to cover your legs either with tights or tracksuit bottoms. I prefer tights worn with shorts outside, because I feel anything else slows me down. However, I am rather open to shouts of 'Go, Superman' and 'Hey, it's Biffo the Bear' and other ridicule, so this might not be the style for you. You can buy tights to match your thermal top; or raid your aerobics wardrobe (so who cares if they're shocking pink?) or simply wear any thick footless tights. If you have legwarmers, by all means use them as an extra layer, either on legs or arms.

Tracksters. A more modest winter leg covering is the tight-fitting, but not skintight, trackster – nylon trousers with drawstring waist and zip legs which go on and off easily over shoes.

Hat and gloves. A large amount of body heat is lost through the head and hands, so you'll need a hat (or hooded sweatshirt) and woollen or cotton gloves. Any hat and gloves will do – you don't have to spend very much on these. I buy cotton sleeping gloves from Boots. If my hands get hot I can tuck them into my shorts and at under a £1 a time it doesn't matter if I leave them somewhere (which I usually do).

Reflective clothing. It makes sense to be seen at night, and you should buy something reflective – either a reflective tabard or the belts that cyclists wear – if you don't have luck in your running or sports shop, try a cycle shop.

Suit yourself

Tracksuits. If you have a pair of tracksters and a supply of sweatshirts you don't *need* to buy a tracksuit as well. Women are wearing tracksuits as leisure gear all the time now – it's nice that we are relaxed enough about our bodies to be able to do so.

Strictly speaking, the purpose of a tracksuit is to keep you warm before and after running when your body temperature can drop quite rapidly. It should be easy to get on and off over shoes. If you actually train in a tracksuit you will need something to change into, or put on top, after your run. Make sure the top and bottom of the tracksuit overlap – if the top parts company with the trousers your midriff can get very exposed!

Rainsuits. If you're not running very far, and you're getting into a hot bath immediately afterwards, getting wet isn't a problem. Synthetic clothes don't hold water as much as cottons so your vest and shorts (in summer) – or thermal top and tracksters in winter – won't become waterlogged. If you're really on a shoestring you can take a leaf out of the experienced marathoner's book and wear a plastic rubbish sack with holes cut for your head and arms – some people have started *and* finished marathons dressed this way! However, a rainsuit both looks nice (some women go shopping in theirs, and you couldn't do that with a plastic rubbish sack) and keeps the wind and rain off your body.

A rainsuit material needs to be light, waterproof, and allow sweat to evaporate from the inside, so that you don't feel as if you're running in a sauna bath. The best is also the most expensive. It's called Gore-Tex, and at nearly £100 a suit is far too expensive for most pockets.

A better buy is the proofed weathersuit, which is lightweight and ventilated and, though it makes no claims to be 100 per cent waterproof, will certainly keep you dry in all but the most torrential downpour.

Possessions

Always carry a coin for the phone – you might twist your ankle or feel cold and need a lift from somewhere. You'll usually need to carry your front door or car keys, and you should always carry some form of identification. What do you do with all your possessions? There are a number of purses available which attach to wrist, shorts or shoelaces, or you can simply bundle your worldly goods up in a small plastic sandwich bag and safety pin it to the inside of your shorts.

For identification you can either wear a dog tag as suggested in Chapter Two, or do what Spence Ingerson has done with her kidney donor card: 'Sign it, cover it with clear plastic on both sides so that it survives being tucked in your shorts when you're out running.'

One last tip – never race in new clothes. Wear and wash them a few times beforehand.

PROJECT 10
THE NEW YOU
Have a photo taken in your new gear and stick it in your Book, or send it round to a few friends who remember you as an ageing fatty. Are you feeling good? You're *looking* terrific!

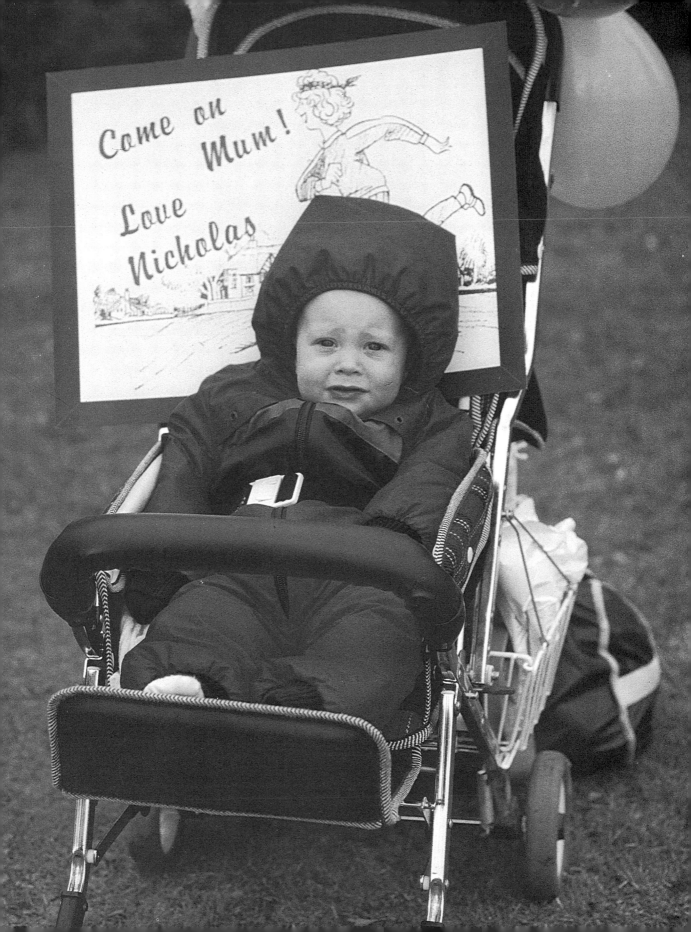